COPYRIG...

But what does that mean?

Throughout the writing process, my goal is to create something worthy of sharing. It's not uncommon to find me laboring over a single paragraph late into the night. With that in mind, I'd really appreciate it if you would kindly ask before using any part of this publication. You can easily find me on Facebook, here's the direct link. https://www.facebook.com/james.lilley.393950. *Thanks.*

TABLE OF CONTENTS

Short Introduction

INTRODUCTION

If you are finding this content for the first time, welcome! Think of these new chapters as stepping stones to healthier lands. They are your shortcut to a less stressed, more energized, healthier version of you.

It's fair to say, this 2nd book in the series covers more topics than a Swiss Army knife. It's actually bursting at the seams with new and engaging content. Some of this information you may surprise you, *some of it will shock you to the core!*

The aim of this book is to turn complex information into something that's enjoyable to read. Often times this book will read like two old friends chatting over a pot of tea. I'll also be striving to keep things real.

Based on six years of meticulous research, this isn't another health book to look good sitting on the shelf. Nor is it intended to replace mainstream medical advice. But rather to be of service as a tool to complement it.

As an added bonus, many of the topics covered inside are interactive. At the end of each chapter, leading health gurus come to you in the form of clickable video links. Handpicked with intent, these short clips help to smooth out the learning process. As well as bringing balance to the many topics discussed. **Fans of Dr. Mercola, Dr. Axe, and Dave Asprey, are sure to find this content enjoyable.**

Here's what a recent reviewer had to say *"As a holistic therapist, I have literally read hundreds of "health" books. None have impacted me as strongly or deeply as this one."* – Sandra Kagan, Ph.D.

Below are a few of the things covered in this book

· How to find a good doctor, and how to avoid the not so good ones

· Learn exciting techniques that most people have never heard of

· Where to find the cleanest foods on the planet without going broke

· Understand why certain foods make you and your loved one's sick.

· Discover simple stress management techniques (that work)

· What to eat and when to eat it, (is Keto the new Paleo?)

· Know which supplements work, and which to avoid

To get the most out of this journey, it pays to bring along an open mind. If you have no room for such mental flexibility then better to leave now, empty-handed. While I'd be sorry to lose you so early, there is peace in knowing that neither one of us is wasting our time. For those who stay, I suspect illness unites us, if only in our vulnerability to it.

In every sense of the word, my style is independent. With no one pulling my strings, I have nothing to fear from telling it like it is. That said, your health is important to me, as it should be to you. What you are about to read is to debated and even disagreed with. And no book can replace working with an informed health care professional. My willingness to share the following disclaimer is an acknowledgment of that.

DISCLAIMER

The statements made in this book have not been evaluated by the US Food and Drug Administration (FDA). The products mentioned in this book are not intended to treat, diagnose, cure, or prevent any disease. The information provided in this book is not a substitute for a consultation with your own physician, and should not be construed as individual medical advice. Although this book contains information relating to health care, the information is not intended as medical advice and is not intended to replace a close person-to-person relationship with a qualified healthcare professional. If you know or suspect that you have a health problem, it is recommended that you first seek the advice of a physician before trying out any medical program or treatment. All efforts have been made to assure the accuracy of the information contained in this book at the time of publication. The author disclaims any liability for any medical outcomes that may occur as a result of applying the methods suggested in this book.

Coming inside?

Amazon
Top customer reviews

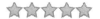

I loved EVERYTHING about this amazing book

I have owned and run my own health food store for over 24 years and this is a book I will recommend to ALL my customers. James is straight to the point and because of his personal health struggles has so much insight as to the REAL issues. Love, love, love this book

Amazon
Top customer reviews

One of the most real and influential books I have read!!!

First let me say I have never read a "health" book before. This was not just a book about someone telling you that you HAVE to live your life a certain way. This book makes you look at everything in a very different perspective. The author brings us into his struggles (which we all have in one way or another) and talks through his book as if he is talking one on one with a friend. This was a fantastic read and I strongly suggest anyone reading it.

Welcome

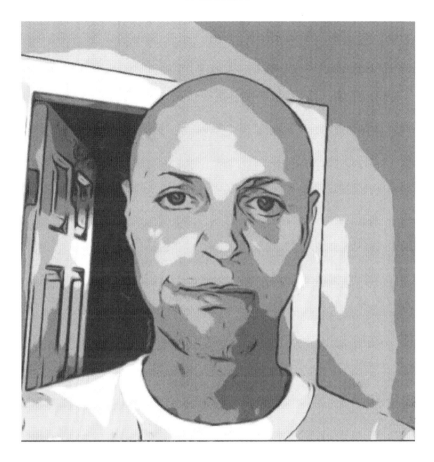

*Like an incessant obsession, this book
has quietly burned inside me.
This wasn't the story I intended to tell,
and yet here we are,
staring each other firmly in the eye.*

Chapter 1

WHY BUY LOCAL?

Back in the day, my grandparents used to own a fruit and vegetable shop in the heart of England. Out of pure economic necessity, what came and went through the front door was either local, sustainable, or in season. At the time, this was just the way food was traded. No doubt, if the shop were around today it would be viewed as trendy or even upmarket. Had my grandad still been alive, I'm sure he would be left scratching his head to know that the organic business model he used out of pure necessity, would today be seen as hipster!

After both of my grandparents passed away, the shop quickly changed hands. Today it sells bargain priced booze and the only place to buy fresh produce is at the giant supermarket down the road. Perhaps as a reflection of our changing times, all the supermarket vegetables come tightly wrapped in plastic. Quite remarkably, it is estimated that those same vegetables will have traveled an average of 1500 miles to get to the supermarket. *I know, right? It kinda makes a mockery of the whole cutting carbon emissions thing.*

To those within the food chain, the words "local and organic" have suddenly become lucrative buzzwords. This is where we pick up the next part of our story.

Bugs eat profits. I know this and so do large-scale organic farmers. Make no mistake, farming is hard work and you can bet anyone getting up at 5 a.m. is in it to make money like everyone else. And to be clear, there is nothing wrong with making money at 5 a.m. or any other time of day. However, if you think all your organic produce arrives on your table pesticide free you would be wrong. Large scale organic farmers aren't about to risk crop failure and certain financial ruin just to bring you a fresh head of kale.

Ever wondered why your organic kale comes to the table without hundreds of tiny bug holes in it? It's been sprayed with an "organic" pesticide. What you need to quickly wrap your head around is that ALL pesticides, organic or not, share a common goal: to repel living things.

Here's where it gets sticky.

According to the USDA, the organic label only restricts the use of synthetic pesticides. Pesticides like copper sulfate and rotenone *are* permitted to be sprayed directly onto your organic produce. *Am I saying don't buy organic?* Nope, that's not what I am saying at all, but some of us have become so desperate to believe in the benefits of organic food that we only see what we want to see.

The aim of this chapter isn't to tickle your ears with sweet words, it's to help you understand the value of clean, local food and show you where to buy it without going broke.

Let's take this a step further by looking at that pristine organic USDA seal of approval. Would it surprise you to know that it can be handed out to products that use only 95% organic ingredients during processing? For this reason, anything carrying the organic label may not be strictly 100% organic.

Look, I'm not shooting organic food down – I'm simply saying that in today's busy world of commerce it pays to be aware that the only truly organic food is home grown. Your next best option is to know the name of the farmer who grows it.

Not all organic food is as squeaky clean as we would like it to be. With that in mind, perhaps some of the smaller local farmers without an organic seal are being harshly overlooked.

The controversy over organic food can begin even before the first seed is planted. Whether or not the seeds are organic means only one thing: that the original seed-producing plant was grown according to organic standards. If a hybrid seed is planted, the resulting plant will still be organic so long as synthetic pesticides and fertilizers aren't used.

To be clear, organic food that's been grown specifically for supermarkets has its place in your recovery. It's a huge step in the right direction and an absolute upgrade of what they usually try to sell us. The point I am trying to make is this: don't be too quick to discount your small local farmer just because he/she doesn't carry that holy grail of organic seals.

Try looking at it this way: there was a time when our ancestors' food was truly organic. Today farmers who choose to grow "organic" food are often shackled in regulation. The irony is those nonorganic farmers who drown our foods with synthetic pesticides are less regulated.

Surely we have this all twisted. Shouldn't the regular farmers who are spraying copious amounts of carcinogenic pesticides on our food be the ones held accountable and buried in paperwork?

Either way, there are times when small independent farmers can't get the organic certification simply because of the added paperwork and costs involved. Fees typically include paying the government for site inspections, application fees, and annual certification fees.

If an organic farmer wishes to conform to all the regulations he/she must find the time to stop work whenever a government bureaucrat visits the farm. If the small local farmer wants the organic seal, he/she is inevitably forced to jump through hoops to get it and in the process loses valuable time and resources. With the small local farmer now squeezed out, I sometimes feel we are a quick to trust the large-scale organic label and slow to ask questions.

As evolutionary biologist Christie Wilcox explained in a 2012 Scientific American article, even "organic" pesticides can be toxic. Copper sulfate, when digested in large amounts, can lead to damage in the tissues, blood cells, liver, and kidneys. While I'm not suggesting toxic levels are being applied, we should be aware of any pesticide that has the potential to cause us harm.

Rotenone is another pesticide sprayed onto organic crops and is notorious for its lack of degradation. Studies show that copper sulfate, pyrethrins, and rotenone can all be detected on plants after harvest. Hmm, I see, perhaps we need ask more questions of large scale farmers, not fewer.

With (or without) the government organic seal of approval, enthusiastic young farmers are the lifeblood of the local food movement. They often bring clean food to farmers' markets and shouldn't be discredited for lack of paperwork.

Diversity in farming is a good thing and relying too heavily on a small number of people for our food should be obvious cause for concern. Many small farmers are the backbone of independent farming and they deserve your support just as much as any large scale organic farmer does.

The goal of this chapter isn't just to get you to buy clean food, I'm asking you to go a step further and know the name of the farmer who grew it! Make a connection with the person growing your food. Small farmers need you to survive and you need them to thrive. Ask yourself, how many of your friends on Facebook are farmers?

Still not convinced, huh?

DESERT ISLAND

Imagine we find ourselves stranded on a desert island with 150 other people and one bag of seeds. Everyone agrees that three things are needed our survival: food, water, and shelter. Fortunately, this island currently has enough coconuts to get us through the first few weeks while the (non-GMO) seeds grow. Unfortunately, nobody seems to have a plan beyond this so the group decides to put YOU in charge of its survival. I know, right? Now we are all up the creek without a paddle.

You quickly realize that you need to make some pretty big decisions. What percentage of this group will you send out to find water? How many do you put in charge of growing those seeds? How many do you put to work building a shelter? If you split the group evenly into 50-50-50, I think you'll eventually be okay.

Even if you split the group 20-70-60 I still think you will make it. However, if you choose to have 149 people sitting around looking at computer screens all day while just one person grows the food, I'll think you are certifiably insane.

How is this relevant?

Well, think about it. Doesn't it make you feel a little uneasy to know that, statistically speaking, the U.S. has just one farmer responsible for feeding 155 people seven days a week. This situation becomes a little more unnerving when you understand that most supermarkets have an inventory strategy called JIT (Just-in-Time).

Supermarkets employ JIT to increase efficiency and decrease waste by receiving goods only as they are needed. Even a small disruption in

14

the JIT supply would see our supermarket shelves quickly stripped bare.

Are we there yet?

No?

Okay, try this. With or without an organic seal, small local farmers have a passionate connection to their land – it's in their blood. Local produce is always fresher from the local farmer and often less expensive. Superstores are now growing at an expediential rate with some of them now opening around the clock seven days a week, taking with them a huge slice of independent pie.

When the purchasing power of superstores is allowed to become disproportionately influential, income is taken away from the surrounding local businesses. When all the small businesses are gone, giant superstores will be free to dictate what you eat so long as it remains profitable for them to do so.

Fortunately, superstores are not the only game in town and you can still find clean food locally in small mom and pop shops or at your local farmers' market so long as we get out there and support them. Buying food locally also gives you the added benefit of buying what's in season and fresh.

Compared to the huge superstores (which never seem to close) small farmers' markets are usually held just once a week, obviously reducing their competitiveness with the bigger players. Unless we get out and support them more, this way of trading food will soon vanish. What's in it for you?

I know you've been paying attention, so you already know the key to your recovery is your gut. It takes whatever nutrients you give it and then loops it back into the cells. Rather than buying your "organic" broccoli from a superstore, when you buy local you actually get to meet the person growing it. Where there is a connection there is also accountability.

Am I saying you have to cut the giant superstores completely out of your food loop? Nope, but it's important we try to adjust the balance by sourcing as much locally grown produce as possible. I get it, waiting once a week for a farmers' market can increase your chances of going without, so rather than complain about it don't be afraid to take a shopping list with you on farmers' market days. *But why stop there?*

Once you have made a connection with your local growers it's totally okay to ask them if you can buy from them directly on non-market days. Often small local farmers will have additional eggs, vegetables, and meat for sale and they may even be pleased that you asked.

This is how food used to be bought and sold. Sometimes you just have to open your mind and be on the lookout for nutritional opportunities rather than following what everyone else does.

NO FARMERS
NO FOOD

Having a thriving farmers' market in every town used to be the norm, but what can you do if your town or city doesn't have one? The most obvious choice is to move. Yup, finding clean food obviously needs to become a bigger priority in your life. Failing that, I encourage you to travel to the next town or to the one after that. You could also think outside the box and approach your local supermarket produce manager and ask if he or she would consider carrying more local produce. This idea supports your local farmer and it may be a good fit for all concerned.

If you still can't find a local farmer, then you could try hooking up with a local gardener. Anyone who grows food for a hobby usually grows more than they need. Generally speaking, gardeners are a pretty friendly bunch and they enjoy doing what they do – it's why they do it. Who doesn't like to have their hobby appreciated?

If your budget is ultra-tight, keep a lookout for garden allotments. This untapped idea can be a nutritional goldmine. This leads me nicely into the suggestion that even if you only have a small window box, you can begin to grow something yourself. This won't sustain you, but it does serve as an important psychological step to get you thinking differently about local food.

> Growing your own food is like printing your own money.
> – Rod Finley

People often complain about the price of clean produce, which is why our ancestors played a much bigger role in growing their own. Today you can still buy a pack of 250 organic lettuce seeds for a few bucks. A single fully-grown store-bought lettuce will cost you more. Lettuce seeds are super easy to grow and even when left unattended they grow like weeds.

The same applies to tomatoes. You really don't need much skill or more than a couple of feet of soil to grow them in. I agree it all takes time, but so does checking your email. Just sayin'.

Once you see how easy it is to grow a few lettuces and tomatoes you may even become bold enough to grow even more things for yourself.

We spend millions of dollars keeping our lawns green, yet you can't eat the stuff and you certainly can't smoke it. Growing something, anything, gets you thinking beyond the scope of the supermarket.

These superstores have become masters of distraction and even with the best intentions we keep finding ourselves going back into them for organic food and leaving with a pair of socks. Think about it, these distractions put your food bill up every time you go to the store.

THOSE DAMNED SWEDISH PEOPLE

Perhaps we need to look at this problem from a different perspective. In Sweden, a small group of city folks took it upon themselves to grow just a few basic vegetables. At the end of the growing season they traded with each other for more variety. It worked out well for everyone involved. So why does this feel so unnatural to us?

A little more food for thought (author knuckle bumps reader for unintended pun): imagine if one day visitors from another galaxy dropped in to visit and began observing those crazy Swedes growing their own food.

They then observed that other group, yup, you know who I mean, the ones being slowly poisoned to death by pesticides. Which group would the aliens regard as crazy? The group of humans working together to grow what keeps them alive, or the group of humans eating out of cardboard boxes while sitting on their excessively manicured lawns?

So, while we are waiting for our home-grown lettuce to come to fruition let's ponder our options. They say the road to hell is paved with good intentions. Promises and plans must be put into action, otherwise they are useless. The way to make this work is to make the small local stores your first port of call and then fill in any gaps at the supermarket. Doing it the other way around rarely happens.
In all sectors, diversity is the lifeblood of healthy commerce; whether you are buying a cabbage or a carpet, small family business owners need our support.

Without economic diversity the world would become a very scary place. I'm reminded of how the Cadbury company once managed to successfully run their chocolate empire with exemplary values. Today? Meh, not so much.

CHOCOLATE

From humble beginnings, Cadbury's chocolate began in 1824 by a family of practicing Quakers. As they grew so did their workforce. As a way of giving back to the local community, workers were taken out of dirty slums and moved into houses built expressly for Cadbury employees in a beautiful village environment.

At a time when many workers were uneducated, Cadbury also built a school for its employees children, and a doctor's office where Cadbury workers could receive free medical care. Mr. Cadbury regularly walked the factory floor and not only knew the names of his workers, he knew the names of their family members. The Cadbury workforce had value and working conditions steadily improved year after year.

Throughout Victorian times, the Cadbury name continued to grow, in part thanks to a loyal workforce. The Cadbury brand prided itself on selling only quality products. As the business expanded, it was suggested that growth could only be sustained if the Cadbury family began to advertise. A meeting was set up and several ideas were pitched to the Cadbury owners.

After several hours, all the ideas were rejected on the grounds that it was dishonest to suggest their chocolate product was better than it was.

Fast forward and today the Cadbury chocolate company is no longer in the hands of the Cadbury family. Instead it was broken up and sold off to shareholders from around the world. I suspect many of those shareholders have never set foot on the factory floor.

While the stock price may have increased in value, the value of a Cadbury worker has never been more undermined. When American food giant Kraft moved in to buy up the Cadbury brand, workers were seen protesting with banners that read, "Please don't sell us out." The value of those workers is now secondary to the profit line.

> Try not to become a man of success,
> but rather try to become a man of value.
> – Albert Einstein

What did we learn from this chapter?

On average, just one farmer is responsible for growing the food of approximately 155 people. Buying local produce in season will enhance your nutritional intake as well as help the local community grow. Small independent shops often have greater ties with local growers which helps keep the local cycle going.

Homework:
- Challenge yourself to know the name of your local farmer.
- Grow one thing from seed and see where it leads.
- See if there's a farmers' market in your area and start going.
- Check out this short video by Dr. Axe.

https://www.youtube.com/watch?v=bMzEbRqWA-k

Chapter 2

THE IMMUNE SYSTEM

In book one we talked a lot about the importance of the digestive system. In this chapter we shine the spotlight on the immune system. When we look at the immune system under a microscope, it's plain to see that *this* system, above all others, is truly mind blowing. Once fired up, your immune system is an equal match for a wide range of would-be enemies.

This formidable system can defend itself from multiple foreign invaders while at the same time launching a counter-attack with deadly precision. To be clear – your immune system comes well-equipped to deal with high level threats on a minute-to-minute basis. For anyone seeking good health, the immune system is your new BF.

But there is a problem, can you see it?

To keep it running at optimal performance levels, the immune system requires key nutrients. Unfortunately, many of these nutrients are now missing from our diets – and in some cases, they have been replaced by toxic ones. *Hmm, I see.*

For some, the immune system has now become a nutritionally downgraded version of its former self making it far more susceptible to illness. Rather than first looking to correct the underlying nutritional deficiency, man has taken to propping up a weakened immune system with a variety of pharmaceutical products.

Make no mistake, good science has an important role to play in fighting disease, no question about it. This isn't a question of being for or against any particular ideology or approach; it's about exploring ways to achieve the *same* goal of fighting disease with an enhanced set of tools.

For the immune system to function optimally, it has very specific nutritional needs. We could just as easily flip that last statement around and say that sugar, in all of its forms, has the potential to *weaken* the immune system. *No really, it's a true.*

> Thinking is difficult, that's why most people judge.
> – C.G. Jung

For the past 100+ years, science has had the unenviable task of trying to rid the world of infectious diseases, often by provoking the immune system. For the past fifteen years, that goal has somewhat intensified, and yet illness continues to thrive.

Science is quick to point out that it doesn't have all the answers, which in turn opens the door for intelligent debate. Perhaps in our relentless pursuit to control disease, we have reduced the risk of one problem, but inadvertently increased the risk of another.

How so?

In case you missed it, autoimmune conditions are now currently skyrocketing out of control, and nobody seems to know why. Perhaps, man's quest to control disease has become a double-edged sword.

> There's more than one way to skin a cat.
> But from the cat's perspective they all suck.
> – Ze-Frank

The definition of an autoimmune condition can be thought of as an immune system that has become confused to the point where it now fails to recognize the difference between itself and extensions of itself. In simple terms, the immune system has been spooked.

Once triggered, a confused immune system can launch an attack on itself anywhere in the body. Rest assured, your immune system is anything but dumb, *so why would it do that?*

When the immune system is treated with well, it becomes a formidable ally, but an immune system that's gone haywire, is a problem that few understand. For now, let's take a closer look at a *normal* functioning immune system.

PAC-MAN

The immune system essentially protects us three ways: by detecting, reflecting, and destroying. It's as if something is lurking deep inside us and playing a giant game of Pac-Man even as we sleep. The skin is our first line of defense and forms part of our innate defense system. It's a living barrier – like a wall built around a castle – and even a minor paper cut will allow you to see a miracle unfold right before your eyes. No?

While science is still patting itself on the back for splitting the atom, your immune system quietly gets on with completing far more complicated tasks every second of every day.

The last time you got a paper cut on your hand, do you remember healing it? Nope, of course you don't because an automatic chain reaction of events unfolded and did all the work for you. While you were wandering around with a flower in your hair your immune system went straight to work within a millisecond of the cut occurring.

Nerves quickly transported a signal directly to the brain that the skin had been breached, the brain then took that information and informed the immune system to be alert and ready. An immediate cascade of healing phases followed as tiny cell fragments sprang into action. Instantly, tiny capillaries contracted to reduce bleeding and platelets keenly meshed both sides of the cut together with speed and precision which helped stem blood loss.

THE MIRACLE CURE

Even though it was just a paper cut, inflammation flooded to the area as those tiny fragments worked diligently on your behalf. But wait, there's more...mast cells automatically joined the fight and began releasing histamine into action. This helped dilate blood cells and increased the flow of blood to the repair site.

Before long, here came the oddly named white blood cells neutrophils and macrophages, working as a kind of tag team to consume bacteria and remove damaged tissue. Once the cleanup job was complete, a signal was sent back to the brain to let it know inflammation could stop.

Now fibroblast cells began to migrate from surrounding tissue secreting collagen and rapidly multiplying as they did. A week later, the scab fell away and you couldn't even see the repair. Your paper cut was fully cured (and that's the only time I'm going to be using the C-word in this book).

That was just a paper cut, and this remarkable chain of unfolding events I've just described is a massive over-simplification of the healing process. It might surprise you to know that the mind-blowing complexity of it all still isn't fully understood by science. Sure, science has given all the main players lots of fancy names like neutrophils and macrophages, but the exact nature of every single reaction remains a mystery (and still amazes).

Sadly, humans have become quick to tamper with the immune system, once the immune system turns rogue on you, doctors are pretty quick to throw up their hands and have little to offer in the way of permanent solutions.
This is the clearest signal yet that the medical system has underestimated the complexity of the immune system and still continues to provoke it. When the only tool being used is a hammer, everything soon begins to look like a nail. I suspect there is more to this debate than meets the eye.

Autoimmune conditions can be notoriously difficult to diagnose and treat – although an autoimmune condition is actually pretty easy to spot. *So how do you know if you have one?*

First, you will feel pretty miserable. Then take a look at your medical file. Have you seen five or more doctors? Is your file as thick as the US tax code and filled with bloodwork tests that have all come back "good"? At home do you have a cupboard full of medicine, but still feel like crap? Do you have a second cupboard full of natural supplements that only seem to make things worse? Adding insult to injury, somewhere along the way has it been suggested that your suffering is all in your mind? And have you remained undiagnosed for at least two years? If this is you, perfect, and welcome to the perplexing world of autoimmunity!

An autoimmune condition can be like having an octopus on your back with its long tentacles reaching into every corner of your body. Whatever part of your body it comes in contact with, it attacks.

This now becomes your new autoimmune condition (or at least label). It's widely believed that once you have one autoimmune condition the chances of getting a second escalate. So, there's the good news out of the way. And now for the bad.

Once you have an autoimmune condition there is no cure for it; once the gene has been switched on it can't be switched off. However, before you throw yourself under a Number 52 bus, let me throw you a helpful lifeline. His name is Dr. Gundy and he is internationally recognized as being an inventor, researcher, author, **and one of America's top certified doctors.**

Dr. Gundy is also one of the early pioneers who have been able to demonstrate with statistical analysis that positive results can be experienced in patients with autoimmune conditions by reducing certain foods from their diet.

This is done in part by making drastic dietary changes that include restricting all grains, dairy (didn't will already cover these?), legumes, and foods belonging to the nightshade family which include foods like peppers, potatoes, and tomatoes. These groups of foods are collectively referred to here as lectins.

Maybe some of you are a little freaked out right now, running around your kitchen muttering random stuff to yourself about not eating lectins. Try to take a deep breath; it's going to be okay, okay? This is all covered in another chapter.

One way to reduce the lectin content of food is to cook those types of vegetables with a pressure cooker. So while there may not be a cure for autoimmune conditions, symptoms can be managed. And the good news is, in the right circumstances this can be done almost to the point where symptoms cause an absolute minimum amount of disruption.

Yes, it takes effort to get there, but what's the alternative, a life of pills and misery? I think we can do better than that. The human body is unlike anything else on our planet and the immune system is arguably the most complex, impressive, and effective system of all; it was put there to protect us. Let's work with it, not against it.

Anyone suffering from an autoimmune condition will typically experience a set of symptoms that reflect an immune system gone totally bonkers and out of balance. Once the immune system gets out of balance, a whole lot of things can go wrong at the same time. In an effort to simplify matters let us now split the immune system into two parts consisting of Th1 and Th2.

Please note, the following information is an oversimplified overview, the opinions in this chapter (as with all others) are for information purposes only, they are not intended to treat, diagnose, or prescribe for any illness or condition. For your specific diagnosis and treatment, consult with your own doctor or healthcare provider.

SO WHAT THE HECK ARE
Th1 and Th2 CELLS?

Th is an abbreviation for T-helper cells which form part of the immune system. Their job is to recognize and destroy any foreign microorganism that can cause disease. Th1 cells typically deal with infections by viruses and certain bacteria.

They are the body's first line of defense against any pathogen that gets inside our cells. Th1 cells tend to be pro-inflammatory. Th2 cells typically deal with bacteria, toxins, and allergens. They are responsible for stimulating the production of antibodies. Th2 cells tend not to be inflammatory. But what does that mean?

Well it may sound complicated but it's really not, just keep in mind that both groups work together, sometimes Th1 may do more of the work and, depending on the threat level, Th2 may play a lesser role. As the threat changes, roles are quickly switched. Once the threat has been neutralized the two stand down and return to equal balance.

In an ideal situation neither one is displaying a more dominant position than the other. This is how a well-balanced immune system should work. However, in some people a prolonged pattern of either Th1 or Th2 dominance occurs. Each can then suppress the activity of the other and problems begin. Why is this important to know?

Think about it, knowing if your immune system is Th1 or Th2 dominant can be a hugely important part of the puzzle because knowing allows you to figure out which is the best course of action to take and which you should avoid. Rather than identifying with an ugly illness label, wouldn't it be better if people had the knowledge to be able to say "hello, my name is Joe and I'm Th1 dominant".. Just sayin.

Remember some supplements have the potential to crank up the immune system. So perhaps now it makes sense why that cupboard full of natural supplements made you feel worse. Anything that boosts one side of the immune system tips the balance. If you have an autoimmune condition, then this has the potential to increase an attack. So how do we know if we are Th1 or Th2 dominant?

Well, as you might suspect there are a couple of clues that we can now explore. There is also a Th1, Th2 cytokine blood panel that your doctor can order.

Th1 cells are part of what's called cell-mediated immunity, which is an immune response that does not involve antibodies but does involve the release of various cytokines in response to foreign proteins. If this problem were a basic image, this is how it might look.

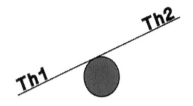

People who are typically Th1 dominant (but not all) may have delayed food sensitivities, increased brain fog, fatigue, increased likelihood of Type I diabetes, multiple sclerosis (although MS can be found in both Th1 and Th2 dominant types), Hashimoto's, Grave's disease, Crohn's Disease, psoriasis, Sjogren's syndrome, celiac disease, lichen planus, rheumatoid arthritis, and chronic viral infections. Again, these are generalizations and as with any autoimmune condition it can easily manifest itself in multiple ways. Hmm, I see.

Being Th1 dominant means the immune system is constantly amped up. Obviously balance is important, but another telltale sign of the Th1 dominant person may be a tendency to catch fewer colds and some reports even suggest lower cancer rates. The flip side is a higher incidence of autoimmune conditions.

Beware of any supplement that has the potential to boost the immune system which could, in theory, increase Th1 and add to the problem. For example, supplements like Echinacea, astragalus, olive leaf, elderberry, and any medicinal mushrooms that are immune boosting.

If you are Th1 dominant, be aware that lots of supplements have the potential to make you feel worse, so remain vigilant as this is by no means a complete list!

Th2 DOMINANCE

Having an immune system that is Th1 dominant is one thing but what happens when things swing the other way? Functionally, Th2 cytokines have effects on many cell types in the body because the cytokine receptors are widely expressed on numerous cell types. Th2 cells stimulate and recruit specialized subsets of immune cells, such as eosinophils and basophils, to the site of infection or in response to allergens or toxins leading to tissue eosinophilia and mast cell hyperplasia. I know, right? Who thinks this way? Let's look at an image of this instead. Ahhh, that's better.

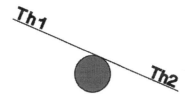

Th2 has some pretty beefy weapons called B cells and antibodies. These B cells are just totally fab to use in battle as they help produce even more antibodies whenever needed and they just keep going and never run out of ammo – cool, right? This is done to ensure there is always enough ammo on hand should any foreign invader ever try to sneak into the body. Also keep in mind that Th2 cells are anti-inflammatory.

Now can you see the importance of balance? Once a foreign invader enters the body it finds itself locked in mortal battle with BOTH elements of Th1 and Th2. As the battle rages, the pro-inflammatory process needs to be "cooled down" using anti-inflammatory cytokines; hence it's a team effort. It's really not helpful having one side that's always dominant because, left unchecked, systemic inflammation could easily occur throughout the body causing untold damage. When inflammation gets out of control you can sometimes smell it under the armpits as a more pungent type of BO. Before you shoot me down for being weird again just think back to the last time you felt really ill, your body had a totally different smell to it, am I right?

When Th2 gets to be the dominant one, we may be more inclined to get seasonal allergies, asthma, food and drug allergies, and anaphylactic reactions rather than systemic inflammation. Th2 dominance can also be caused by a variety of issues such as heavy metals like aluminum, mercury, and lead which are known to lower immune function. Hello again, heavy metals – haven't we met before?

When the immune system is shifted too much to the Th2 system, people generally have less inflammation but their potential to develop allergies to everything increases. It's the allergens that then begin causing problems.

Other possible diseases linked to Th2 dominant conditions may include Lupus, allergic dermatitis, atopic eczema, sinusitis, inflammatory bowel diseases, asthma, allergies, colitis, and multi chemical sensitivities. Some reports even suggest an elevated Th2 may increase the risk of certain cancers. Either way, once the immune system gets stuck out of balance, we lose. I know, right? Let's not go there, let's instead focus on solutions. Agreed!

Interestingly, Lyme disease has the ability to throw Th1 out of balance because Lyme disease creates a state of perpetual Th1 dominance;

this unfortunately results in constant inflammation, causing an ongoing downward spiral of damage in the body.

Because Th1 dominance is pro-inflammatory, perhaps now we see the importance of eliminating all those foods that create inflammation. Foods like sugars, foods loaded with preservatives, refined and fried foods, and fast foods all contribute to complicating the problem.

Do you see how this is all beginning to fit together? Spices like curcumin, turmeric, and ginger along with omega 3 oils are thought to be helpful because they may help counteract inflammation imbalance.

Th17

In this chapter I've strived to keep the complex simple; however the immune system is a vast subject and we didn't even get chance to talk about Th17 cells. In case you are wondering why, it's because they are a subset of activated CD4+ T cells that are responsive to IL-1R1 and IL-23R signaling. I know, right? Just thinking about it gave me a headache too.

However, if the whole Th1, Th2, Th17 concept has piqued your interest then be sure to check out a website by the name of self-hacked.com. There you will find a formidable amount of solid information that you are unlikely to find anywhere else.

Autoimmune conditions are tricky and you may benefit from someone who thinks outside the box. Fortunately, the person behind the self-hacked blog (Joe) has the advantage of looking at the problem with fresh eyes. I greatly admire the good work Joe does and I read his blog often. If you visit his site please tell him I said hi.

LYMPH

The design of the human body is as incredible as it is complicated and it's difficult to fully appreciate or cover every aspect of it in one book. However, I would like to briefly mention the lymphatic system which is a network of tissues and organs that help rid the body of toxins, waste, and other unwanted materials.

The primary function of the lymphatic system is to transport lymph, a fluid containing infection-fighting white blood cells, throughout the body. Under each of your armpits are more than twenty tiny lymph nodes.

These small but highly sensitive lumps act like checkpoints. If we know the lymphatic system's job is to help fight infection, you have to question the logic of squirting antiperspirant in such a delicate area. When you stop to look at the loooong list of toxic ingredients (which usually includes aluminum), it makes me wonder why some people choose to sleepwalk into illness this way.

As the name suggests, antiperspirant stops your skin from perspiring by literally clogging it up. Seeing how the skin is alive and needs to breathe, perhaps applying an antiperspirant isn't a smart idea for anyone looking to overcome illness. The irony is the more we overload the lymphatic system the worse B.O becomes.

Unlike the heart, the lymphatic system has no pump and requires movement to push lymphatic fluid around the body. This fluid moves best when we move, which is bad news if we happen to be sitting still most of the day with toxic chemicals under our armpits, but good news if we commit to moving more by either walking or jumping on a trampoline. Hippocrates said it this way: "Walking is man's best medicine."

I've never actually read any of the James Bond books or seen any of the movies but I do know plenty of people who have. Apparently, if you are fan you will already be aware of the "James Bond shower." Maybe Ian Fleming wrote about this technique to show Bond's brave Scottish ancestry, or maybe he was just trying to keep the character healthy. Either way, a James Bond shower is highly effective at moving lymph and pretty easy to do. I know you are going to love this one!

If you haven't been moving around too much then neither has your lymphatic fluid which is a shame as all that junk is now sitting in your trunk. However, all is not lost! Hop into a hot shower and relax – feels good, right?

Now at some point simply turn the water all the way to cold and count to thirty, longer if you can stand it. Repeat this three times and it will really help push the lymphatic fluid around the body. Doing this every day is no guarantee that you will live longer, but by the end of the week it will seem as if you already have!

What did we learn from this chapter?

When the immune system can no longer cope with the demands placed on it, the potential for it to spiral into the complex world of autoimmunity increases. The immune system is far from stupid – perhaps we have inadvertently tricked it once too often.

The human body is indeed a complex marvel, but we are not the grand masters of the universe we'd like to think we are, and yet we remain hell bent on trying to harness the complexities of the immune system. Too often we fail or make things worse. I'm just sayin, perhaps there are better ways to enhance the immune system, for example by first removing the burdens we place on it and then flooding the cells with key nutrients. Personally, I also find an occasional teaspoon of colloidal silver is helpful with infections, along with optimizing my Vitamin D levels.

Homework: if this chapter struck a chord with you, then take the time to research whether you are Th1 or Th2 dominant. You can do this with an initial scoping of symptoms followed up with a blood test.

You can also check out Joe at self-hacked, as always please feel free to mention where you found this information. Here's the direct link: https://selfhacked.com/

Chapter 3

A WALK ON THE DARK SIDE

We humans like to think that we are the one's running our own bodies and yet we have this strange system lurking inside us that has the power to shut us down without ever asking our permission. While it's true that we can override our need for sleep with stimulants, sooner or later the body will always have the last word. No?

Let's see, who's really in control, you or your body – ready? Try staying awake for seven nights in a row. Meh, didn't think so, perhaps we are being outsmarted by ourselves with good reason.

Sleep is essential to good health, no question about it, and better sleep quality equals better productivity. On the flip side, lack of sleep can adversely affect the way we act and feel. Reasoning quickly becomes impaired, attention to detail is lost, and even problem-solving skills decrease.

These are some pretty big clues that sleep is important to us, and yet so many of us try to fight going to bed at a reasonable time. The aim of this chapter is to help you appreciate the value of your sleep and also to help you improve it. Let's go take a look under the hood.

Despite comprising only two percent of the body's weight, the brain gobbles up a whopping twenty percent of your daily energy intake! Make no mistake – your brain is a big fat an energy hog. Each night when you go to sleep, a cleanup crew gets to work and literally washes the brain to ensure that everything is ready for the next day.

It does this by using cerebrospinal fluid which moves through the brain along a series of channels that surround blood vessels. Cerebrospinal fluid is a clear liquid that surrounds the brain and spinal cord.

This process is managed by the brain's glial cells. Science defines this as the "glymphatic system" which helps remove a toxic protein called beta-amyloid from brain tissue. OMG are you getting this? Beta-amyloid is renowned for accumulating in the brains of patients with Alzheimer's disease!

BRAIN DRAIN

From the moment your life began, your body has been using sleep to recharge and repair. We don't need to fully understand the mystery; we just need to know that sleep is yet another tool we can tap into to assist in our recovery.

Think of it this way: we are quick to understand the importance of recharging our cell phones every night, yet we fight the same simple logic of getting enough sleep to recharge our bodies. The human brain is infinitely more complex than even an Apple iPhone, so it's hardly surprising that our brain fails to work when we suffer from lack of sleep

TICK-TOCK

Every evening when it begins to get dark outside, our brain begins increasing its production of the hormone melatonin which makes us feel sleepy. Melatonin production is designed to be switched off again upon sensing the morning blue sky. This is how we evolved. It's important to understand this because so much of our lives are now affected by the invention of the electric light bulb which gives off a blue light similar to the morning sky.

This manmade blue light can really throw our sleep into total chaos. Keep in mind that altered melatonin levels can lead to an increase in depression and irritability. Sabotaging your sleep with any form of blue light is easy to do. You can do it by playing video games, watching TV, or even looking at your computer screen. Your body is programmed to go to sleep when it gets dark outside and blue light totally messes up that whole process. I accept that I'm not your mom and you can go to bed at whatever the hell time you like, but it's smart to begin winding down at least two hours before bedtime rather than playing Grand Theft Auto V1 until the minute you're ready to close your eyes. Just sayin'.

If you want to be a successful sleeper, challenge yourself to become a total blue light Nazi. Remember, sleep is important, otherwise the body wouldn't force us shut down and do it every night. Light streaming in through a bedroom window is something else to think about. Street lights, car headlights, and even the moon can all affect your sleep quality. For better sleep, quality black-out curtains are essential.

Waking in the middle of the night also poses an interesting problem because if your eyes see a bright light, your chances of going back to sleep are affected. Keep in mind those harsh bathroom lights will really disrupt melatonin, so wherever possible try to tone everything down by using small plug-in type night lights.

Tip- You can limit the amount of blue light that's being emitted from your computer screen by installing a free download called F.lux. This tracks the time of day in your time zone and as evening comes on gradually reduces the amount of blue light on your computer screen. It may seem a little odd at first, but it can serve as a helpful reminder that really you should be winding down. If you decide you don't like it, simply uninstall it.

If you find yourself waking up in the middle of the night because you are hungry it could be a sign that your blood sugar isn't being regulated properly. If this is you, try eating a bowl of rice an hour before bed as rice is pretty slow to digest. If rice isn't your thang, try a teaspoon of raw local honey at bedtime instead, why? As you sleep, the brain still uses energy and does so by tapping into glycogen which is a form of sugar stored in the liver. If you try this route be sure to use only quality honey. Much of the honey found in the supermarket is imported from China; it's simply not the same standard as raw local honey and results will differ.

If you drink coffee, keep in mind that it can stay in the system for six or more hours, even longer in sensitive people. Try not to drink alcohol in the evening. Initially it may help you feel drowsy, but it will prevent you from entering the deeper stages of sleep which is where the body does most of its healing.

Many of us have heard that we need a standard eight hours of sleep, but it's the quality of sleep that's important. I'd like to suggest that we all have different needs, some of us may do better on six hours of sleep and others may need more. Ever wonder why teenagers always seem to need more sleep? The teenage years are a critical time for brain development so it's unfortunate that teenagers, who have the most need for sleep, are often the ones who don't get enough.

Perhaps we should be encouraging them to sleep in more, not less. If you are a teenager, show this book to Mom; if you are a mom, let your teenager know this isn't an excuse to stay in bed all afternoon, it's a suggestion that she or he should be going to bed at reasonable time. Somewhere, there is a compromise and a little give and take is sometimes helpful. Perhaps trade an early night off the computer for a few hours extra sleep in the morning…. just sayin'.

If you live to be seventy-five, you will have spent, on average, twenty-five years of your life asleep. Ever wonder what happens in sleep?

When we lie down and close our eyes our brain rests and our heart rate slows. This restorative and relaxing part of sleep helps induce the NREM (Non-Rapid-Eye-Movement) sleep cycle. NREM sleep is then followed by the REM cycle (Rapid-Eye-Movement). Research has shown that REM is the part of the sleep that helps consolidate our emotions. This is also the cycle where muscles relax but the brain is in full activity.

As the name suggests, REM sleep is where our eyes begin rapidly darting back and forth. In this state, brain waves are most similar to our waking hours. This is deep sleep, but in order to get there two things must happen. We need dark and we need quiet. Darkness helps with the production of melatonin and quiet just because I said so.

If sleep has been disrupted for any length of time, try not to take anything that might spook the system after 6 p.m. In sensitive people, certain medications and even supplements can really throw the system off.

I'm really not a fan of pharmaceutical sleeping pills as they can leave a person feeling groggy throughout the following day. Even worse, drug dependence can become a problem down the road. If you need a little extra help to fall asleep try the following.

MAGNESIUM

Sustained levels of stress will often deplete magnesium levels and if our goal is to experience better sleep then magnesium is your friend. Magnesium is used by the body as a currency for more than 300 enzymatic processes.
Today it's not uncommon for people to have a magnesium deficiency. When this important mineral becomes depleted it can produce a wide

range of serious ailments ranging from anxiety to cardiovascular disease.

However, before you head off to the pharmacy to buy a bottle of magnesium pills know that magnesium isn't absorbed very well through the digestive system. The better way to get magnesium into the system is by combining both oral and transdermal methods. Transdermal simply means that it is absorbed through the skin.

SALT AND SODA BATH

To increase your magnesium level and help you sleep better, it may help to try a "salt and soda bath." To do this, simply pour two cups of a quality Epsom salts into a hot bath one hour before bedtime. The heat will allow the Epsom salts to be absorbed through the skin and thus flood the system with magnesium sulfate. Add the same amount of Arm & Hammer baking soda to the water and this may help drain the lymphatic system and balance your pH. Some reports suggest that a Salt and Soda bath may even be helpful to decrease radiation levels from x-rays – but that's a whole other story.

If salt and soda baths aren't your thing, you can also buy transdermal magnesium online and regularly apply to the skin throughout the day and then monitor how you feel. If the magnesium is of good quality, you can also expect to have more energy during the day and feel less stressed at night. Yup, magnesium really is that cool.

NIGHTMARES

If a lack of sleep has been an ongoing issue for any length of time a sense of bedtime anxiety may soon develop. In more extreme cases, a set of recurring nightmares may set in. Yup, been there done that.

While there could be many reasons for your recurring nightmare, I have at least one theory and a very simple way to test it. First, throw ALL your pillows in the garbage. Why?

In good health our immune system is able to deal with toxins quite well. When we are stressed/not sleeping properly the immune system becomes over-taxed and less efficient. Most pillows have fire retardant added into them, some more than others. Flame-retardant resembles the molecular structure of PCBs, which have been linked to reproductive problems, impaired fetal brain development, and even cancer! Is flame retardant enough to cause nightmares in those with a weakened immune system? I believe so. If nightmares have been a problem for you and you want to put my theory to the test, seek out a set of less toxic pillows. If you are on a tight budget, just try switching out your pillow for another brand and you might just get lucky.

Without wanting to sound like a hippy, you could also add a few drops of lavender oil directly to your new pillows. This will further aid relaxation and help reduce that nighttime sleep anxiety. This can be particularly helpful with kids, if you want to upgrade your sleep try buying an oil diffuser. These things work great, although it might take a couple of consecutive nights before you see the full effect.

CBD

If you are still struggling to sleep, here's another tip you can try. CBD oil may prove much safer than sleeping pills. CBD oil is taken directly on the tongue at bedtime and it gently eases us into sleep.

A wide range of new studies offer supporting evidence of other benefits of CBD oil, one exciting new area even relates to children with uncontrollable epilepsy. In this area, CBD oil appears to be working where conventional medications have previously failed. In today's homework assignment you will find a short TED talk that will change your perception far beyond anything I can write. I'd really like for you to see it.

CBD oil currently has scientists all over the world keenly researching its many benefits, CBD oil has zero funky effects and it's quite an ignorant statement to suggest that it has. For your peace of mind and my amusement, I would encourage you to research this in more detail but try not to be too freaked out by one word. That word is cannabis, I know, right? We've reached that point. However, you should know CBD oil cannot in any shape or form get you high (sorry if that disappoints some of you).

CBD oil is a legal derivative of cannabis; however, CBD oil can only be sold with the TCH component extracted. TCH is the part of cannabis that's sought after by people who are looking for a high. To be absolutely clear, CBD is a world apart from this. Again let me stress you cannot get high from CBD oil.

BETA-1, 3D GLUCAN

If CBD oil still sounds a little too rock and roll for you then I can totally respect that and perhaps I haven't explained it well enough. If this is you, then maybe we could try something a little more traditional that's backed by research from prestigious universities around the world.

With more than fifty years of research behind it, Beta-Glucans are arguably one of the most studied naturally derived supplements on the planet. Like so many other effective compounds, Beta-Glucans isn't a one trick pony.

Beta-Glucans have a wide range of other benefits. According to research carried out by Dr. Vaclav Vetvicka Ph.D., Beta-Glucan 1, 3D even has some exciting cancer fighting benefits. However, in this chapter we are looking only at its effectiveness as a sleep aid.

It's worth mentioning that Beta-Glucans work as immunomodulators. This simply means it helps restore balance to the immune system. Think Th1 and Th2 imbalance from the previous chapter. Again, don't be in a rush to overload the body with too many things at once and be sure check with your own doctor before trying anything new.

With Beta-Glucans you tend to get what you pay for and the brand of Beta-Glucans I like best is sold by Transfer-Point. It's a little more expensive than other brands but you may find it helpful. I have no affiliation with this company (or any other). If price is an issue, first try some of the less expensive brands. If you see a positive result from the less expensive brands then more power to you.

Sometimes it can be helpful to switch things around from week to week but it's important not to try too many things at the same time because doing so has the potential to make sleep deprivation worse. But a little trial and error should put you on the right track.

Tip – There are lots of herbs to help you sleep and my personal favorite is chamomile tea. If you have one, make the tea in a small hot flask and let it sit overnight, I find that steeping the tea for this length of time seems to increase its potency and you have the tea already made.

Another sleep idea to try is a grounding pillowcase. You can find these online. The pillow connects to the earth supply in your home and it can help to calm the mind. For it to work your home needs to properly earthed, you should test this before buying the pillow.
This can be done with an inexpensive tester from any DIY store; it's a light-up device and costs around five bucks. This concept of grounding is covered in more detail later.

There are plenty more sleep tricks to try, but rather than overwhelm you, remember that using too many sleep aids at the same time is counterproductive. We covered a lot of ground in this chapter so let's quickly recap. Keep your sleeping quarters cool, quiet, and above all else dark. Limit all blue light in the evening and perhaps even try eating some rice for supper. You could also try CBD oil or Beta-Glucan but try them on separate nights. Chamomile tea is best steeped and a salt and soda bath works well for some people.

Lastly, the mattress you sleep on plays a huge role in your sleep. I recently purchased a new mattress from Purple.com, so far I've been pleased with it. If you are in the market for a new bed be sure to check them out.

What did we learn from this chapter?

Without sleep life quickly becomes dull and stressful. Sleep is an essential part of living which is why we typically spend a third of our lives doing it. Blue light at night is a huge problem as it throws our whole system out of whack.

Homework: Below is a real moving video clip by a dad with a pot-taking eleven-year-old daughter. *I know right, but this talk is well worth watching and it will totally challenge your perspective.*

https://www.youtube.com/watch?v=3N8QMeIsX2c

Chapter 4

THE GOOD THE BAD AND THE UGLY

It's fair to say that my own brush with the US medical system left room for improvement, although I refuse to be jaded by the whole experience. I don't believe any doctor goes to work with the intention of damaging a person's health. Certainly there are plenty out there who go to great lengths to improve the quality of their patients' lives; we should all be extremely thankful to have them. To be clear, **I'm glad to report that good doctors and good nurses save lives.** But that's not to say *all* doctors hit the same high standard.

When it comes to broken bones, gaping wounds, heart attacks, or any type of sudden trauma the work a doctor does is nothing short of miraculous. These dedicated men and women deserve the highest credit and we should salute them for the brilliant work they do. Clearly, there are plenty of good doctors who listen to their patients and can swiftly bring about good results – top marks to all the good doctors out there. Let's not forget the army of diligent nurses and paramedics who also deserve out upmost respect.

However, when symptoms present themselves in a vague fashion the medical profession can at times fall short of our expectations. Diseases such as chronic fatigue, crippling anxiety, and devastating depression are examples of this. And cures for even the common cold and cancer remain elusive.

The same would apply to a whole bunch of debilitating autoimmune diseases whose root cause are often written off as either "unknown" or genetic. Once labeled, these types of illnesses remain shrouded in mystery – although, I have my own theories on the subject.

So while it's fair to say that good people exist, the law of averages dictates that in any profession there will be a percentage of average people working right alongside the more excellent ones. Depending on the intensity of your desire to get well, you may find average results frustrating. The gold standard for finding a good doctor is simple: if you are getting good results then you have a good doctor. If you are getting average results, then you are being treated by an average doctor and a rethink is in order. If you are getting very poor results ...well, that's not hard to figure out.

In a perfect world all doctors would be perfect, but doctors are not gods and with more than 400+ US doctors committing suicide every year let me assure you, they are just as human as you and I. Sometimes they get it right and, unfortunately, sometimes they get it wrong. If for any reason you feel unhappy with the results you receive from your doctor, then for God's sake don't be afraid to speak up. It's also important to note that good doctors and nice doctors are not always the same thing. Here's a true story...

A friend of my family has been dealing with a health issue for the past year or so. She has worked in the medical industry most of her life and has a great relationship with the doctor treating her. It's obvious that she likes him a lot and she is now trusting him with her life. However, it's plain to see that twelve months into her illness, her progress has been stagnant at best. A more critical mind might suggest she has actually gotten worse.

Maybe we all see things differently, but to me, being treated by a "nice" doctor can become a real drawback because the only thing that really matters is results. Having been locked into a likeable doctor for almost a year, this lady has little more to show for it than polite conversation and a series of inconclusive blood tests. Given the current health of the nation, I fear this same scenario is being played out across the country.

Average doctors have become far better at public relations than they are at treating people. We would do well to keep firmly in our minds that any doctor we employ is there to fix a problem. As in this case, finding a doctor you like can be a real disadvantage. If your goal is to get well, you may need to look past the polite BS and cheery bedside manner and find someone with a proven track record of bringing solid results to the table. Even if that means you don't necessarily like the person or their methods.

BLOODWORK

Bloodwork certainly has a place in medicine and has been shown to uncover a whole range of potential problems, but this is just one tool and it should never override a patient's physical symptoms. Today we appear to have this seemingly obvious truth a little twisted. Medicine now relies heavily on computerized blood tests and apparently nobody has the time to listen to the patient describe his or her symptoms. During my own brush with illness my wife once pushed me into the doctor's office in a wheelchair to discuss my bloodwork. After several minutes the doctor looked up from the paperwork and with a smile and announced that my bloodwork had come back "fine."

Personally, I don't believe any doctor goes into medicine with the intention of making mistakes, but I was very obviously NOT fine. I felt like grabbing him by the lapels and screaming "LOOK AT ME, I'm sitting in a wheelchair, you idiot! Do I look fine?" To rely so heavily on bloodwork alone displays an absence of sound reasoning. It also begs the question, if blood tests are so effective why are so many people still plagued with illness?

In days gone by, old-school doctors leaned toward asking a series of probing questions and then listened carefully to the answers. Today a computer is quick to churn out numbers based on averages. Essentially, a blood sample is attempting to make a match with a patch of dry ink. This arrangement may work well for the computer, but let's not forget that we are humans, and our variables are often incalculable.

The number a computer spits out for a 6' 5" man with green eyes shouldn't be in the same range as for a 5' 2" man with only one eye. You catching my drift?

Am I saying blood tests have no place in medicine? Nope, never did say that. I'm saying it is imperative that you find a doctor who listens to you. Yes, blood tests are a useful tool but only when used in conjunction with a little common sense. If a patient looks unwell and says he is unwell then you would think that any blood test to the contrary should be questioned. But today we seem to have that basic concept all backwards.

Consider this: Addison's disease is a serious complaint relating to the adrenal glands. In order to diagnose it a doctor can order a blood test to measure levels of sodium, potassium, cortisol and ACTH. So far so good, and to be fair this test is effective at measuring these kinds of levels. If the blood test picks up the symptoms of Addison's, bravo to the blood test, you win.

However, early stages of the disease are often missed, especially if the patient isn't probed for information. While the blood test does well to pick up a full-blown case of Addison's, it does little to notify either the patient or the doctor in advance. According to the test's logic, one day you don't have it and the next day you. Voila!

For sure, all things must have a starting point and maybe the symptoms of adrenal fatigue are an early indication of adrenal dysfunction. But as with leaky gut mentioned earlier, the medical

51

profession doesn't recognize adrenal fatigue, so it doesn't have a conclusive blood test, much in the same way that leaky gut doesn't.

Again, I 'd like to stress that bloodwork can be a valuable tool. The point I'm trying to drive home is that heavily relying on a blood test and ignoring the patient has the potential to bend all the laws of common sense, and in doing so does a great disservice to the patient.

Tip- If you find that progress with your regular doctor is has become stagnant you may find it helpful to search for someone who practices "Functional Medicine." Functional Medicine leans toward addressing the whole person, as opposed to an isolated set of symptoms.

LOOKING FOR A USED CAR?

When we're looking for a reliable used car we expect to do our homework. We may even cross-reference prices and like-for-like MPG ratings. Some of us may even bring into question the car dealer's past integrity. To find that perfect used car we may diligently pump our friends and family for recommendations, yet when a car breaks down the only thing we stand to lose is a little money. It would seem logical that whenever we seek the services of a doctor we should practice at least the same level of diligence we do when making a used car purchase.

If you have an illness, finding a good doctor is a smart first step in the right direction, but this shouldn't mean you are ready to hand over full responsibility after a brief fifteen-minute appointment. A motivated, informed patient should be able to spot an average doctor from a mile away and that can mean that he or she will recover much faster.

I'm rarely impressed with the bricks and mortar of a doctor's office, the fancy artwork and certificates on the wall or the pitch perfect classical music being piped into the waiting area. Rather, give me a doctor who can answer the "Why am I ill?" question.

We live in a digital age with information all around us. If you have a medical appointment coming up, use that time to educate yourself. Going into any new situation blind and expecting a positive outcome is nothing more than hopeful. Prior to your appointment take notes and have a series of questions on hand.

This is your life and if progress has been stagnant then you need to become an active player in your own recovery, if need be, fight your own corner, don't just sit there blindly following the instructions of others in the hope that it's all going to work out for you. Come on now, deep down you know I'm right. If you want to get well stop being a tourist in your own recovery. Now is a good time to stop taking a back seat with your health and instead slide into the driver's seat and grab the wheel.

DEATH

It's worth noting that the tools of a doctor's trade are often steeped in profit. For sure, medications and medical procedures have the potential to save lives but, as I've learned (to my detriment), they are not without risks. The term medical malpractice is one we should ALL fear because it is now a leading cause of death in the U.S. If we break down that statement it simply means this: we go to the doctor, he or she gives us something for our illness, we take it, and we die.

No?

Okay, check this out.

In 1999 the pharmaceutical giant Merck released a drug by the name of Vioxx. With a TV budget running into the millions, Vioxx quickly became one of Merck's bestsellers. Americans were prescribed Vioxx as an aspirin substitute because it was believed to produce fewer complications. I know, right? What could possibly go wrong?

By 2007, thousands of people had died and the class action suit that followed was eventually settled for $4.85 billion. Unfortunately, cashing a check from inside a casket is a trick I have yet to see done. But wait, there's more. By the time Merck paid its fine, it had technically made more profit from selling a deadly drug than it had paid in fines! Conservative figures suggest that Vioxx killed hundreds of people, if not thousands, and yet nobody went to jail. What's up with that?

> Our prime purpose in this life is to help others.
> And if you can't help them, at least don't hurt them.
> – The Dalai Lama

The real concern is that Vioxx was first put on the market in 1999. Despite early alarm bells ringing and vigorous claims that thousands of patients were experiencing deadly complications, Vioxx remained on the market right up until 2004!

"First do no harm" is a noble oath that good doctors aspire to; it's also the same one many of those doctors prescribing Vioxx took. Perhaps doctors' iconic white coats should be required to carry the names of their sponsors the way NASCAR drivers do. To expand on this point we could easily fill up the remaining chapters with other deadly examples of pharmaceuticals gone rogue, but I suspect you have already been conditioned to accept that side effects are a necessary evil. This is often done with great skill via the medium of television. Shall we take a look?

MAN BOOBS

For the past decade or so I personally haven't owned a TV set nor do I want one. Whenever I happen to catch sight of someone else's TV set

I am literally stunned at the misleading images some drug companies will use to bait and sell their products. The carefully staged slick image of a healthy looking fifty year old man running through a sun-drenched sprinkler system on a manicured golf course rarely suggests that the product being marketed to you has a list of potential side effects that include death. How is death even a side effect?

Even if you live to tell the tale, some of the side effects from these drugs can be darn right strange. Recently I overheard a legal commercial asking the following question, "Have you or your son developed breasts from taking the drug Risperdal?" Maybe a more accurate picture would be to have the same healthy looking fifty year old man running in slow motion through a sprinkler system while wearing a double D sports bra. Just sayin'.

The irony is this: had a vitamin company sold any type of supplement that suddenly gave fathers (or their sons) boobs, the FDA would surely have them hanging upside down in jail faster than you could say Wonderbra. For some pharmaceutical companies with a stock price shooting through the roof, this appears to be just the cost of doing business.

Maybe it's me, but if a prescription drug gave me (or my sons) boobs as per the legal commercial, I'm not sure I'd be sitting patiently around on my sofa waiting to be told my next step. Make no mistake, I'd be banging on the doctor's door and shouting, "Come out and see what you've done, you idiot!"

Is this a good time to mention that doctors used to promote cigarettes on TV?

Doctors were once so keen to have us smoke, they were happy to appear in TV commercials to help us understand the health "benefits" of cigarettes. You can still see some of these old commercials on

YouTube. Seriously, you kinda gotta see this level of arrogance to believe it. For "proof" of no adverse effects, check out this link:
https://www.youtube.com/watch?v=TOKc6TNwlj4

Today we can look back at their pro-smoking statements and ask, what the hell were they thinking? Ever wonder how future generations will judge this moment in history?

In the right hands, a good doctor can be a blessing, although it does seem a little bizarre that most of us will spend more time researching a vacation than we do a medical procedure. Unless we play an active role in our own health we are giving total responsibility to someone else.

Let us be clear, when it comes to dangerous side effects, we are the ones left to pick up the pieces. Most people who become ill go to the doctor to get healthy. In my case, it happened exactly in reverse. Then I had to fight long and hard to regain my health on my own. A little backward, don't you think?

So, if you already have a good doctor and effective medications I congratulate you; this isn't always an easy combination to find. If this route is working for you, I again urge you to continue. All that matters is that you find a way to get well, how you get there is of little consequence.

LEGS

Clearly things can and do go wrong with medical procedures, but for this next example imagine for a moment you woke one morning with serious pain in your left leg. Over time this pain worsened to the point where you began limping. As the pain intensified a friend quite rightly suggested that you see a doctor. The news you received from the doctor is damning; tragically the doctor informs you that amputation is the only course of action.

Despite reassurances that prosthetics have come a long way you are deeply reluctant to cut off your left leg. On the way home your leg is hurting like hell and deep inside you accept that the doctor is right – obviously that leg needs to come off.

A month or so later you find yourself back in the doctor's office flipping through a glossy prosthetic leg magazine. After filling out the paperwork you are relieved that a date has finally been set for the operation. Now imagine waking up from that same operation and seeing your idiot doctor holding up your right leg. Yes, he amputated the wrong leg. True story.

In 1995, Tempa surgeon Dr. Rolanda R. Sanchez of the University Community Hospital listed the wrong leg for amputation. He and his lawyer Michael Blazicek publicly presented their side of the story.

Personally, I would have thought it a difficult case to defend once exhibit "A" (the leg) was presented, technically leaving him without a leg to stand on, so to speak. Whoa! I'm just telling it like it is.

As for the patient, God only knows what he must have been thinking as he faced the unenviable decision of having to decide for a second time whether or not to have his left leg cut off.

But every cloud has a silver lining. The next time around we can safely assume that the chances our patient's correct leg will be cut off are as close to 100% as anyone could hope. Easy now ... or would you rather I just deliver your medical news in a dull format?

You might think this is an isolated incident and you would be wrong. It is well documented that removing the wrong limb – and even the wrong organ – happens with disturbing regularity. During seemingly routine operations there have even been reports of medical instruments gone missing and turning up stitched inside the patient! My point is this: don't settle for average, do your research, be informed, fight your own corner or live with the consequences. Rushing into a relationship with a very nice but "average" doctor allows for ample opportunity to repent at leisure – but that's not what you're after when you seek medical help. So please, if you are heading for a hospital, have good people around you and remain vigilant; it's important to play an active role in your own recovery.

HAPPY NOW?

If cutting off the wrong leg reeks of incompetence, then this final example suggests arrogance. A former neighbor of mine takes care of her disabled son. She has done so lovingly and around the clock for more than eighteen years. One of the problems she frequently faces is that he goes into seizures. Her son has been on medication his whole life and after this many years, Mom has become quite proficient at understanding the benefits and limitations of his medication.

A new doctor came to town (always a red flag) and during a routine visit he suggested giving the boy a much higher dose than he'd been taking. Mom told him they'd tried this in the past and it only made the problem worse. The doctor totally ignored her and persisted and the mom, feeling pressured by the expert, finally caved in. Out of fear of getting into trouble herself, she followed the doctor's orders. Retelling the story with tears in her eyes, she told me that the same afternoon the poor kid went into one of the most violent seizures she had ever seen. She immediately called the doctor. Only this time it wasn't to seek more advice at this turn of events, it was to say, "Happy now?"

I'm sure a good doctor would have listened to her eighteen plus years of first-hand experience and employed a degree of common sense, but all too often we allow ourselves to be intimidated by a seemingly educated person. Deep down we all know when something doesn't feel right, but we allow ourselves to be swept along without questioning because nobody ever told us that it's okay to say no.

When faced with ANY invasive procedure first do your homework, speak to people who have been in your situation (and in this day and age that's easy to do). Then compare their results with your expectations. People are always in a hurry to recommend nice people, but we should remember that we aren't looking for nice, we are looking for competence and results.

Ultimately it's always going to be your health that's on the line. Hear me now, if something doesn't feel right with any procedure, speak up for yourself and politely but firmly say no. It's your body, which means you don't even have to explain yourself. You should never feel pressured to do something that makes you feel uncomfortable just to make someone else feel comfortable.

HOW TO FIND GOOD PEOPLE

Going into ANY doctor's office lacking awareness will leave you with no way of knowing if you are being treated by a competent doctor or an average one because both will appear the same. Good doctors aren't always the most expensive, nor do they need to have the best bedside manner. They do, however, have to have one dead giveaway.

Good people are busy people, and that's okay if he or she brings results. Try to keep this in mind. If you can pick up the phone and see the doctor (or dentist) the same afternoon, that should immediately be a red flag. Most competent doctors will be booked solid as good news always travels fast. If you can get in to see your doctor at the

drop of a hat, then perhaps you should wait for that other guy –
obviously this is subject to your appointment not being an
emergency. (And of course, if the receptionist says, "Wow, what luck,
we just had a cancellation a few minutes ago – otherwise it would be
three months before I could get you in" … well, that too is a different
story.)

This same logic can be applied to anyone who has the potential to
adversely affect your health. Let's take dentists, for example. There
are good dentists and there are average dentists. An average or not-
so-great dentist can have a serious effect on your health with the
potential to last a lifetime. These days most dental practices have
more than one dentist on duty in the office. If you really want to
know who the better dentist is, ask the receptionist which dentist has
the longest waiting list? If your situation allows it, wait it out for that
person. Visit the dentist twiddling his thumbs at your peril.

Had I had the benefit of my own advice earlier I could have saved
myself an awful experience. In poor judgement I took the first
available dentist appointment and my teeth have never fully
recovered. The truth is that dentists have ample opportunity to cause
lasting problems to your health. As mentioned in an earlier chapter,
BPA (Bisphenol A) is the same stuff everyone is freaking out about in
plastic bottles. It should, therefore, be on your radar when the dentist
comes along and wants to put that white plastic filling in your mouth.

Remember earlier when we learned that silver fillings can be just as
problematic. Yup, the name is a little deceptive as a percentage of
that "silver filling" can be made of mercury. I know right WTF? (Why
These Fillings?)

Once a silver/mercury filling becomes an integral part of your mouth,
you can look forward to a lifetime of potential issues. Dr. Chris Shade
Ph.D. has a substantial amount of time invested in this very subject.

His findings are jaw dropping and I would strongly urge anyone with these types of metal fillings to listen to what he has to say in some of his free YouTube videos.

> It is not often that nations learn from the past,
> even rarer that they draw the correct conclusions from it.
> – Henry Kissinger

Sadly, it is still common practice for silver/ mercury fillings to be touted as harmless by some ignorant dentists. Remember, it wasn't that long ago that doctors were keen to have us line our kids up on the street and have them sprayed with DDT! (I am not kidding.) Today we know DDT to be a highly toxic substance and the practice is banned.

Root canals have been known to solve one problem (an abscessed tooth) but create another of equal complexity. Root canals can harbor insidious bacteria because once the inflected the tooth is sealed, it's essentially shut off from the immune system. There are times when it might warrant removing the offending tooth altogether. Bottom line: research any and all medical procedures. If you are happy with what you found, then go for it.

> The doctor of the future will give no medication, but will interest his patients in the care of the human frame, diet and in the cause and prevention of disease. – Thomas Edison

If you find yourself looking for alternative ways to ease what ails you, remember the rule: good people usually stay busy. And this rule applies to naturopaths and/or chiropractors as well. When the spine is out, the whole body suffers and any good chiropractor knows this. Over the years I've met many chiropractors and it's been my experience that most do stellar work. Am I giving all chiropractors the green light? Hell no! I've met at least one who shouldn't be allowed anywhere near the human frame, so as always, if something doesn't seem right to you I urge you to always go with your gut instinct. Sadly, this is a valuable tool that we rarely employ.

A good chiropractor will always use his ears before his hands. If you are in good hands a trip to the chiropractor shouldn't be painful. A skilled chiropractor will fix your problem; a bad one can make it worse. Don't be shy about asking friends or family for their recommendations. Having spent the last ten years living in New England, here's mine.

If you find yourself in Northern New Hampshire, my recommendation would be Dr. Dean Powell of Powell Chiropractic. Dr. Powell is everything a good chiropractor should be. If you find yourself over the line in Vermont, you would do well to check out Lyndonville Chiropractic.

Tip –For any guy who carries his wallet in his back pocket, here's a simple tip that might save you a chiropractic problem down the road. Know that each time you sit down your wallet causes your spine to be slightly out of line, over time this can become an issue especially if you are sitting for long periods during the day. A much better option is to carry your wallet in a front pocket, where it's also less likely to be stolen.

Let' s recap. The goal of this chapter was to guide you into the hands of good people and perhaps even make you smile occasionally in the face of adversity. Before going for ANY medical procedure it's important to do your homework. As an informed patient you can then automatically look forward to a higher standard of care.

Whenever you meet your primary caregiver be polite and respectful but don't be afraid to ask probing questions. Pressing people for the cause of your illness allows you to evaluate that person's understanding of the problem. Without knowing the true cause, any treatment is speculative and has the potential to become detrimental.

This approach should be applied to anyone who comes into contact with your health, be it a doctor, dentist, chiropractor, or any type of naturopathic practitioner.

And finally, I'm often left in total awe at the intricacy of the human anatomy, I really am. I have a reverential respect for the fine detail and complexity of it all. However, it does seem that the older we get the more likely we are to put something "out" as I did recently while working in the garden.

Now you dunnit.

Is it me, or is the design of the spine perhaps a little too intricate? Don't get me wrong, if you are a thirteen year old gymnast looking to do a backbend then it's hard to improve upon the idea of lots of little bones all working together, but for the rest of us? Meh, I think we could do away a whole bunch of them.

As an avid gardener, it seems to me that the spine is sometimes a little too fancy for its own good. I wonder if we could get away with having just one big bone, much as we have in the femur? As long as I could bend up and down when I'm planting my lettuce seeds, I really wouldn't even care if I looked like one of those wooden dipping duck toys. I digress.

What did we learn from this chapter?

The right doctor can be a godsend, but choose your new doctor/dentist with same care you would choose a new (or used) car, and always do your homework. A good doctor/dentist/chiropractor will never feel threatened by an informed patient. Ask questions and listen carefully to their answers. And make sure they are listening carefully to what you are telling them.

Homework: find a good doctor to have on your team. If your circumstances allow it, you may find it helpful to search for someone who practices "Functional Medicine." As always, do your research so that you are certain you are in good hands.

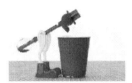

(Couldn't resist)

Chapter 5

THOSE TRICKY TRIGGERS

Some foods have the potential to heal; others can cause negative reactions in some people. The latter are sometimes known as "trigger foods." The time between consuming a trigger food and having a reaction can vary quite a bit, often times there is a mental disconnect (or, there is no immediate obvious connection) between the food and the reaction. The aim of this chapter isn't to give you a long list of what not to eat – it's to make you aware of what those potential trigger foods are.

This doesn't mean all the foods mentioned here are going to be a problem for you, it simply means as you read through this chapter you will be better informed and able to recognize patterns if and when they arise. Don't lose heart – all these problems have solutions. When we learn to recognize the connection between food and the way it makes us feel, it quickly becomes an empowering tool.

From the get-go let's kick off with the most obvious. The Big Four to be on the lookout for are always going to be gluten, dairy, eggs, and nuts. Having this vital piece of information at the very beginning of this chapter will serve us well as we move forward. It also pays to be on the lookout for bad fats, which we'll cover in more detail later. Better buckle up, some of this information gets a little bumpy. Okay, here we go.

Before illness came to pay me a visit, my diet was at best average. I guess I'd always been one of the lucky ones, I had an immune system that worked just fine, which meant I could make dietary mistakes and get away with it. However once my health was sent over a cliff, that was no longer true. I quickly went from never having any type of seasonal allergy or food sensitivity to being confronted with an absolute tsunami of them. I know, right? What's up with that?

To my horror, suddenly many of the foods I had eaten with impunity my entire life were now acting as springboards for new symptoms. Once the immune system becomes spooked, one man's food can quickly become another man's poison.

One of the frustrations I faced was trying to find accurate nutritional information. So often it felt as if the target I was desperately trying to hit was frequently moving. It really doesn't take much to find yourself wading knee-deep through a sea of conflicting misinformation. One day carbs are good, the next they are bad, yada, yada, yada.

It's not that the majority of dietary information out there is incomplete, contradictory, or wrong – the problem is we are all so different. With so many human variables it's impossible for one diet to fit every person. Unfortunately, this fundamental concept is something even the standard food pyramid fails to take into account.

Once you see the problem from this perspective the subject of nutrition begins to make more sense. Obviously there are some BASIC rules that apply to all of us. But the clean fuel your body was designed to run on is likely not going to be identical to that of your neighbors. The world has successfully evolved by utilizing the skill sets of uniquely different people. Perhaps Mother Nature intended food to be used as diverse fuel. How so?

During our early history, the nutritional needs of a hammer-swinging shelter builder would have been very different from those of person who spent most of his or her time trying to solve more complex problems, like inventing a wheel. Today we still have a need for that diversity; we need farmers to grow food, carpenters to build things, engineers to design things, and academics to teach us stuff. Here we begin to see the bones of the problem. Throughout history, no single diet has ever suited everyone.

ORGANIC TRIGGERS

As surprising as this may sound, many of the known trigger foods are perceived to be healthy. Some of them might even be growing in your very own vegetable garden! For that reason, it's important to note early on that even organic food can act as a trigger and with the same intensity as its nonorganic version. I'm not intentionally trying to rain on your vegetable parade here, but unless we are aware of this going forward, then everything else will be built on sand.

Once you have a basic understanding of what these potential food triggers are, the exploding minefield of nutrition becomes a little easier to navigate. I know what you are thinking because I've thought about it too - why would a super smart immune system react like this to healthy food. Right?

In short, a spooked immune system can label something you just ate as a foreign invader. Sometimes this reaction is serious, immediate, and obvious, and sometimes it's less obvious. To describe this reaction, the health industry often uses terms like food intolerance, food allergy, and food hypersensitivity interchangeably. This is not just deeply confusing, it's incorrect.

Food intolerances are relatively common and are said to affect one in five of us. Although reactions can vary, the immune system is not involved in food intolerance. Trying to replicate a reaction to a known food intolerance can be inconclusive because there can be any number of factors contributing to the intolerance. Food intolerances are known as non-immunological reactions.

By comparison, food allergies or hypersensitivity to a particular food are both reactions to a protein found in certain foods. This does involve the immune system. This type of reaction is less common and is believed to affect one in fifty of us.

Once the offending protein has been identified, a predictable reaction can be replicated. With some degree of certainty, even a small amount of food will cause a reaction by the immune system. These types of reactions are known as immunological reactions.

WHY NOW?

Once the body has labeled a particular food as problematic, antigens are made that ignite the immune response. Antibodies that bind to those antigens are then formed. With so much ground to cover, what-say we avoid turning this into a stuffy old science lesson and instead think of this whole process as the body tacking a bunch of yellow sticky notes onto any foreign invader it deems suspect? The body does this as a way to help guide an attack by the immune system. That being the case, and since we know immune system is far from dumb, why would it suddenly begin doing this in relation to food?

Due to the complexity of the immune system, that's a pretty big question to grapple with. To briefly recap, the immune system is highly intelligent and very much alive; it's arguably the most complex, impressive, and effective system of all. Its primary function isn't to find ways to annoy you. Its intent is to protect and yet humans insist on provoking it, perhaps to the point where it becomes totally confused.

Once the immune system is spooked, food sensitivities may be the tip of the iceberg. A confused immune system that has trouble distinguishing parts of itself from foreign invaders is better known as an autoimmune condition. A reaction could manifest itself in a wide range of problems from general fatigue to an outright attack on organs or joints. I know, right? Always a bummer.

To add to the problem, the word "food" has become a loosely a defined term. A spooked immune system then has the unenviable task of trying to figure out which of the 3000+ food additives are friends or foes.

The scope of the problem obviously magnifies when eating out because you really have no control over someone else's cooking. Remaining blissfully unaware or choosing to ignore food allergies, food intolerances, and hypersensitivities can potentially ratchet up the immune response and, over time, provoke a stronger reaction.

For now, let's for a moment step back from the complexities of the immune system and simply agree that the human body is an absolute wonder, and in order to function optimally it requires fewer toxins and more clean nutrients to burn as fuel.

As a rule, anything you can't pronounce on a food label should be an instant red flag. When addressing the issue of food sensitivity, food triggers, allergies, etc., it's vital to cease consuming products that come to you in a box, can, or packet. Yup, we keep coming back to it, food that's packaged gets complicated.

The more complicated the food, the more potential there is for an adverse reaction. Be aware that today many food additives, preservatives, and antibiotics are finding their way into the meat supply. For that reason, it's important to steer clear of the deli counter (or anything else that's been through a meat grinder) because these meats can be loaded with things that are known to trigger a reaction.

On the surface, a simplified diet may appear more basic and for sure this is how our ancestors used to eat long before supermarkets helped make us all lazy and sick. Simplifying the diet is particularly helpful in the early days when flare-ups from trigger foods are more noticeable. Again, not all food reactions are instant; and relief of symptoms doesn't happen overnight.

This disconnect in time can make it harder to find the original source of the problem – not every reaction to food has us rolling around on the floor in anaphylactic shock. Fortunately, solutions are forthcoming when we learn to pay close attention to those subtle signals all around us. Changes in the skin such as excessive dryness, eczema, or itching can be noticed. When a food is the cause of eczema, topical creams are often ineffective.

While these types of symptoms may be viewed as annoying to the host, they also help bring awareness to a wider problem that maybe you can't see. It's as if the body is trying to grab your attention by saying, "Hey, pay attention to me, what you see on the outside is also happening inside." If you suspect something isn't right, try seeking out a good doctor for allergy testing.

Tip - When the eczema creams fail, you could try cutting a thin slice of raw ginger and rubbing the clean side directly onto the area. Obviously, for a longer term solution, try switching to a simple diet.

Any food that causes a reaction will send out a few clues along the way. Skin issues and other symptoms may rear their ugly heads as well as bloating, long-term flatulence, chronic fatigue, and inflammation. Prolonged inflammation is believed to play a role in cardiovascular diseases, autoimmune conditions, numerous cancers, and even diabetes – just to name a few.

Some food excitotoxins like glutamate and aspartate can give the brain a source of excitatory neurotransmitters adding to the cycle of anxiety and depression. Given that psychiatrists receive little or no nutrition training, this important connection can easily be overlooked.

According to Felice Jacka, the president of the International Society for Nutritional Psychiatry Research, "A very large body of evidence now exists that suggests diet is as important to mental health as it is to physical health, a healthy diet is protective and an unhealthy diet is a risk factor for depression and anxiety."

TRIGGERS SIMPLIFIED

To help us better understand this concept we can separate trigger foods into easy to understand groups. All the following food groups mentioned here are heavily steeped in well-documented scientific data. I'm not bringing this information to your attention to intentionally piss you off; it's simply to make you more aware of potential problems.

Finding those elusive solutions becomes easier once we see the fuller picture. With that in mind, try to use this chapter as a guide. If you suspect you are reacting to any type of food, then you are encouraged to research each of these subjects in more detail. Here we go, ready?

First off, let's establish a few ground rules. Any food known to trigger a reaction can also have a foot in more than one food group. I know, right? What does that mean? A simple example of this would be the potato. It's a vegetable, it's a starch, and it's a carbohydrate. At this stage it's not important to know what these different groups mean because they are covered in more detail later. What is important to understand is that the potato (like so many other foods) is capable of belonging to multiple groups.

To help simplify this concept, picture yourself as being a member of a tennis club and a garden club. Even though you are a member of two different clubs, you obviously remain the same person. To take this a step further, we could also say that in addition to being a vegetable, a starch, and a carbohydrate, this active fellow we know as the potato is also a member of yet another club called the nightshades. This is an important group of foods to be aware of because they can be particularly problematic. Here's why.

NIGHTSHADES

In certain individuals, foods belonging to the nightshade family are thought to weaken the tight joints in the small intestine which causes tiny food particles and excrement to spill into the bloodstream and trigger an adverse reaction and increased inflammation. Symptoms may include (but are not limited to) joint pain such as arthritis, fatigue, and muscle pain and tightness. Are you catching this joint pain sufferers?

So why would nightshades foods do this? To better understand this, know that you aren't the only one who likes to eat – so do bugs. Nightshade plants already know this, but they can't exactly pick themselves up and run away to keep from being eaten alive. So they evolved, and to protect themselves from bugs they have developed the ability to produce small amounts of reactive chemicals. Some people will react to these chemicals more than others.

So now that we know that the potato is in this group, you might be wondering what other foods are too. Am I right?

There are more than 2000 plants in the nightshade family. Yikes. Thankfully, the list of the ones you might want to eat is relatively short.

- Tomatoes
- Tomatillos
- Eggplant
- White Potatoes (but not sweet)
- Goji Berries
- Peppers (bell peppers, chili peppers, paprika, tamales, tomatillos, pimentos, cayenne etc.)
- Tobacco (some people chew it)

If you want to see positive results, eliminating foods in the nightshade group isn't something you can do halfheartedly. Why?

Once the immune system has been spooked, it's automatically on red alert. This means you can't cheat even a little bit. Everywhere you go, so does your immune system. An easy self-test is to stop eating all nightshade fruits and vegetables for 30 days and monitor how you feel.

The good news is if you fully commit to cutting out these trigger foods don't be surprised to find that after just thirty days, even those joint pain symptoms quickly subside. While some people have no problems eating foods in the nightshade family they can present problems for anyone with any type of autoimmune condition. This is something to keep in mind particularly if you don't feel well after eating. Unfortunately, foods that are capable of triggering an adverse reaction aren't confined to the nightshade family. As we have some ground to cover let's leave nightshades for the moment and take a closer look at food mold.

MOLD

Most of us are exposed to low levels of food mold at every meal. This type of mold isn't as obvious to the naked eye as is the mold we are used to seeing grow on bread. In sensitive individuals, repeated exposure to an undisclosed food mold can make the diagnostic process all the more challenging, hence awareness once again becomes your key.

In certain individuals, low level exposure to food mold can present itself as headaches or brain fog, higher levels can result in more serious problems. All foods can be susceptible to these molds and there is currently a school of thought that suggests that a peanut allergy may in part be due to the mold found on peanuts. While the nut debate remains speculative, I thought it an interesting addition to the subject.

With so many everyday foods prone to mold, even coffee can become a culprit. It might surprise you to know that EU countries, South Korea, and Japan have strict regulations regarding levels of mold found in coffee; the U.S. and Canada have no such limits. If you are a coffee drinker, where your coffee comes from is important and it's obviously something we are going to look at in more detail later.

LECTINS

Although you may not have heard of lectins, scientists have known about them since 1884. Lectins are found in abundance in certain fruits, vegetables, beans, nuts, legumes, milk, and members of the nightshade family (hello again).

Lectins (not leptins) are a type of protein that can bind to cell membranes. They are sugar-binding and become the "glyco" portion of glycol-conjugates on the membranes. Lectins can be extremely problematic for anyone with a suspected autoimmune condition. There are literally thousands of versions of lectins and not all of them are truly problematic, but some are capable of causing irritation to the gut lining. The worst offenders, deemed to have vastly higher lectin contents, are listed below.

Obviously try to keep in mind that some people are more likely to have sensitive reactions than others. With lectins, these reactions can be widespread and far reaching. Mother Nature devised lectins as a way to allow certain fruits and vegetables to defend themselves against the microorganisms and insects intent on eating them. Lectins help the seed part of the plant survive.

In most cases, seeds can be notoriously hard to digest. They are constructed that way to ensure that when an animal eats the fruit or other plant its seed will later be pooped out intact, thus allowing a new plant to grow. For that reason, if you are going to eat any type of edible seeds it's probably best to soak them until they sprout a tail, which will help with digestion. All seeds aside, some fruits and vegetables have a much higher lectin content than others, and the genetic engineering of some plants may cause some fluctuations. Gee thanks.

In susceptible people, lectins are thought to wreak havoc in the gut by causing spikes in inflammation and a general degeneration of the lining of the gut. A confused digestive system runs parallel with a confused immune system. Dr. Gundy, the director of the International Heart and Lung Institute in California, believes autoimmune conditions such as rheumatoid arthritis and lupus are greatly helped by restricting the overall amount of lectins we eat. For sure, Dr. Gundy is one smart cookie. He has also written several books on the subject. And he has plenty of interesting YouTube clips. If you find yourself leaning toward the autoimmune camp it might be worth taking a look.

Foods with lower levels of lectins include mushrooms, broccoli, onions, bok choy, cauliflower, leafy greens, pumpkin, squash, sweet potato, carrots, and asparagus, as well as berries, citrus fruits, pineapple, cherries, and apples. You can also add to this list animal protein from fish, seafood, eggs, meat, and poultry, as well as fats from olive oil, avocado, and butter – all of which have low levels of lectins.

FOODS HIGH IN LECTINS

- All grains and cereals
- Nightshades, including tomatoes, peppers, potatoes and eggplant
- Gluten from wheat, rye, barley, malt and maybe oat because it can cross contaminate during processing
- Beans and legumes, including soy and peanut. Cashews are considered part of the bean family
- All dairy, including milk, cheese, cottage cheese, yogurt, and kefir
- Yeast (except brewer's yeast and nutritional)
- Fruits should be restricted during the first 30-day trial period and then gradually reintroduced

The good news is you can reduce your overall lectin intake by cooking with a pressure cooker. This method of cooking will help lower the overall the number of lectins in your foods. Moving along nicely, let's take a look at our next trigger – grains.

GRAINS

Grains are found in everything from pasta to spice mixes, cakes to processed meats, and even salad dressing. The list is impossibly long so it's important to note that grains can be found in just about any subset of food. Because of the way grains are stored when harvested, they can also be susceptible to hidden molds. In certain individuals, any grain can become a problem but the one most talked about is the one I'm sure you have already heard of and that is gluten.

While some people may believe that going gluten-free is some kind of new fad, the discovery of this problem grain was actually first made in Holland by professor Willem-Karel Dicke back in the early 1950s. As many already know, gluten is the seed of wheat and an insoluble protein composite. In plain English, this simply means it's difficult for the digestive system to break down. If I were a betting man (and I'm not), I'd be tempted to bet that grains are, at least in part, contributing to your symptoms.

As set out earlier, intolerance to gluten isn't the same thing as an allergy. An intolerance is the lesser of the two evils and it can certainly rear its head in any number of ways. But comparing a gluten intolerance or sensitivity to an allergy is the equivalent of comparing a very bad sunburn to a third degree burn. Obviously, you wouldn't want either, and to the person dealing with it on a daily basis neither illness is desirable. My point is that they are as different as Donald-T and Malcolm-X … just sayin'.

A true allergy to gluten becomes a more serious autoimmune condition known as celiac disease. This results in damage to the small intestine whenever gluten is ingested. For some, the problem with grains goes beyond gluten.

The most common mistake people make when they are told they have an issue with gluten is they wander around the supermarket loading up on bags of gluten-free breads, gluten-free cookies, and other gluten-free snacks. But, wait, that's good, right? Meh, not so fast.

Once you have a problem with gluten you have a spectacularly higher probability of reacting negatively to other grains. Simply switching to a different grain that doesn't contain gluten is no different than switching to a different pack of cigarettes – they are equally bad.

Some people have an immediate and noticeable reaction to gluten; others have a delayed reaction that can occur gradually over several days. This type of disconnect is obviously more challenging to deal with.

If you suspect you have a problem with gluten, the easiest way to test it is to go totally grain free for thirty days. After thirty days, carefully watch what happens as you reintroduce grains into your diet. Yup, you could also get tested by your doctor, but any treatment is going to involve a strategy of total avoidance.

You might wonder why gluten is suddenly getting so much heat when bread clearly dates back to biblical times. That's a nicely thought of question and I'm going to award you five points for effort, but if you are thinking of wheat as being three feet tall and blowing gently in the wind think again.

Sadly, those types of romantic golden wheat fields are long gone and have been replaced by a much smaller, genetically modified version. This type of wheat is often soaked with a broad-spectrum systemic herbicide known as glyphosate (Roundup) and is designed to produce higher yields rather than higher quality. Is it me, or is Roundup beginning to cause more problems than it was intended to solve?

We could easily fill up the rest of this book talking about problems relating to glyphosate and gluten, but for simplicity's sake, let's agree that for some, gluten avoidance has the potential to bring huge health benefits and its worth trying for thirty days. Try to keep in mind that gluten can hide in anything that comes to you in a box, a can, or a packet. It can even be in salad dressing!

To do this right, you need to stop looking at this as being gluten-free and go completely grain free. This is the single biggest reason people with a gluten problem fail to see progress. Until then, you may find it

79

beneficial to avoid all types of grains, especially wheat, corn, barley, oats, rye, and rice.

Tip – To help you on your way, check out a book called Against all Grain by Danielle Walker. It's packed with good ideas and healthy recipes.

MILK

As discussed earlier, there are many reasons why milk can cause problems, even milk from grass-fed cows. In part it may be because the protein component of milk (casein or BCM-7) or the milk sugar (lactose), are not well-tolerated. And remember, cheese and "healthy" organic yogurts form part of the same problem. However, casein and BCM-7 are largely absent in butter made from cows raised in open pastures and generally doesn't seem to pose as much of a problem to those who are sensitive to milk.

CHECK IT

Below is a list of foods believed to cause approximately 90% of all food allergies. Take a look and ask yourself which of these foods you consume on a regular basis?

Wheat and other grains with gluten, including barley, rye, and oats
- Milk and milk related products, yogurt, and cheese
- Eggs
- Peanuts (prone to molds)
- Tree nuts, like walnuts, almonds, pine nuts, brazil nuts and pecans
- Soy
- Fish (mostly in adults)

- Shellfish (mostly in adults)
- Food additives

Just about everything leading up to this point has looked to remove stressors from your body. Bacterial, viral, and parasitic infections are all known to induce or worsen symptoms of food sensitivities, mainly through the mechanism of molecular mimicry. Hence, previous chapters in this book have looked to eradicate them.

Finally, I'd like to invite you take a moment to hear the story of a one woman's recovery which was helped in part by avoiding certain trigger foods and replacing them with key nutrients.

Terry Wahls was a patient with a chronic, progressive disease and found herself confined to a wheelchair. As a qualified doctor, she used all her medical connections to the fullest. Even so, her condition got steadily worse. - Well that's new.

In desperation, she tried a new path that included nutrition and – can you believe it? – today she walks freely. Coming from a doctor I found her particular TED Talk fascinating and it's in today's homework.

What did we learn from this chapter?

Our individual needs cannot be measured with a single diet or blanket approach. Once you have a spooked immune system, the funky world of food can become an exploding minefield. To complicate matters, some of these trigger foods are often perceived as being healthy organic foods.

Homework: listen to Dr. Terry Wahl's TED Talk. If you are reading the paperback version of this book, a simple Google search will take you there, https://www.youtube.com/watch?v=KLjgBLwH3Wc

Chapter 6

SIMPLY SIMPLIFY

In the last chapter we learned about some of the foods you may need to avoid. Solutions to those problems are coming, but for now let's keep things interesting by switching gears and looking at something new. Of all the recommendations offered in this book, the ones in this chapter are probably the easiest to implement and I hope they will make the biggest difference to you and those around you.

Our perception of success is often judged by the number of dollars we are prepared to exchange for each measured unit of toil. We then exchange a percentage of those dollars for material things. More than ever before, the retail industry is keen to help you do this. Gone are the days where we needed to physically stand inside a store. Today, online shopping brings the store to us at any and every hour of the day or night. We can literally shop till we drop while still in our PJs. Left unchecked, this has the potential to become a huge problem. How so?

As it turns out, your financial health, your mental health, your shopping health, and your physical health are all closely connected. The mind tells money what to buy and the body gets to tag along for the ride. So where has the mind been going and how does that affect your health?

$

Well, in this day and age that's actually pretty easy to find out and you need only click one button. Take a quick look at your browsing history over the last twenty-one days and see what it says about you. Tracking your browsing history is sometimes described as a tool "to enhance user experience," others call it "data-combining." Either way, it also doubles as a way to constantly monitor everything you view, and does so with astounding efficiency. Somebody, somewhere obviously wants that information.

Why?

In a word: money – and lots of it. It's a scary thought, but you already agreed to this intrusive monitoring the moment you clicked that "I accept" button without reading that long list of terms and conditions. Don't panic, nobody ever reads that stuff because we all need our internet access at any cost, right? This is not just an attack by those annoying pop-ups ads. Once your computer has you all figured out it works on learning what you are going to buy, perhaps even before you do. When it learns to cater to your spending habits, money (yours) usually flows in one direction, out.

No?

Okay, if you feel that your spending habits are not being directly influenced by the internet then take a look at your credit card statement over the past two months. Hmm, notice it forms an alarming correlation with your browsing history? Sheer chance? I think not.

You are being gently encouraged to buy more things whether you care to admit it or not. Okay, so even if this is true how does owning more stuff fit in with my health? Well, stuff is just stuff until money changes hands and then it turns into pollution. We all like to drink clean water, breathe fresh air, and look at the big blue sky, right? But there's another problem and it goes by the name of stress.

It's an illusion to think more money automatically equals more happiness. Once self-value comes from owning more stuff it can quickly lead to a never-ending cycle of want. The more we have the more we want. Left unchecked, this line can easily become unhealthy and blurred. If we aren't careful, the things we own begin to own us!

Think of it this way: if a news flash suddenly came on the radio and said you had just fifteen minutes to evacuate your house, what items would you throw in your suitcase? Now ask yourself, what could you gladly leave behind? Perhaps we don't need as much stuff as we think we do.

Over the years I've met with some incredibly wealthy and interesting people, some of whom are used to seeing more money in a day than many of us will in earn in our lifetimes, and yet many of those people were unhappy beyond description.

There's nothing wrong with being wealthy or wanting a better quality of life, but we have to be careful that wanting it (or having it) doesn't take on a life of its own. Many of us have been led to believe that luxury is a standard worth chasing after, yet it also has the potential to bring the most stress.

A preoccupation with accumulating more luxury "stuff" can become a trap that tends to lead into a downward spiral of self-inflicted stress. Somebody somewhere will always seem to have more, and yet this thirst for material things steals the one thing we need more than anything else – our inner peace.

Give a man a million-dollar house and it isn't too long before he's peeking over the garden fence at the sixty-foot boat his neighbor owns. The problem with this concept is twofold. First, you should know the definition of a boat is a hole in the water that must constantly be filled with money. Second, nobody cares.

Simplicity is the ultimate sophistication.
– Leonardo da Vinci

Throughout this book I have strived to be upfront with you. To be honest, there was a time in my own life when I too was a dollar-chasing victim. I followed the herd and drove my overpriced pretentious car and even bought the gold Rolex to match, but no matter how hard I worked it never seemed enough. Some twenty years later, wealth no longer impresses me. I find genuine contentment looking at a full woodshed knowing that I have enough fuel to see me through the coldest of winters. To me this has a real and tangible value beyond money sitting in a bank. Today, I really don't care what car I drive, but I do pay close attention to what food goes on the end of my fork.

> A man who views the world the same at fifty,
> as he did at twenty has wasted thirty years of his life.
> – Muhammad Ali

I once sat on a plane next to an elderly Irishman who had a twinkle in his eye. At some point he and I could hear the couple behind us arguing about money. This elderly fellow turned to me and in the softest of Irish accents said, "Son, in this life you can be sure of this, if a man has a wife or a set of wheels, he's heading for problems." In a crude sort of way, he was right, stress does indeed come from two things, the people we surround ourselves with and the things we own.

It's estimated that in a lifetime, the average American will purchase his or her way through a cool 2.7 million dollars' worth of stuff. If owning more stuff enhances your life, more power to you. But take a look around, how much of that "stuff" is really making you happy or has it become like a ball and chain around your neck?

Ever notice how some of the brightest smiles seem to come from people who live in remote parts of the world and who have the fewest possessions. What's really going on here? Why are they so happy and how does this affect our health?

It seems odd that many of us drive around with more spare change in our cars than some people live on per day, and yet somehow we still manage to go into debt to buy more things. According to American credit card statistics, in 2015 the average US household carried $15,675 in credit card debt and $132,158 in total debt.

That's a lot of stuff, and potentially a whole lot of stress. People now own so much stuff they can no longer fit it all inside their houses. It has to be stored out in a shed, over in the barn, crammed into the attic, stuffed in the basement, or taking up all the room in their garage. And when all those places are full, the trend now is to rent a storage unit! FFS how much stuff do we really need?

YOU DON'T NEED MORE SPACE
YOU NEED LESS STUFF!

As I write this, Black-Friday has just come around and I happened to see on YouTube some of the scuffles that break out when greed sweeps the mind and flat screen TVs go on sale. Even though I don't own a TV myself, I fully appreciate that some people like to watch TV. But still, it's hard to imagine what TV show warrants such acts of aggression. Maybe Black-Friday should be renamed Black-Eye-Friday. Although I offer no proof, I suspect it could even be the Jerry Springer show those folks are in such a desperate rush to watch... Jerry! Jerry! Jerry! .. just sayin'.

I get it, people want to save a buck or two on Christmas presents, but greed can soon become a bottomless pit with a deeply repulsive element to it. Wait a second, didn't Gordon Gekko, the lead character in the classic movie Wall Street, once tell us that greed is good?

Huh ... really?

With rising sea levels and darker environmental skies, maybe that classic line from Wall Street should have been replaced with the following quote from Seneca: "The highest wealth is the absence of greed."

This planet that feeds you, your children, and your grandchildren can sustain all of us – it just cannot sustain the current level of consumerism. It's estimated that a truckload of plastic is dumped into the sea every minute of every day. If we continue buying cheap imported plastic at the current rate, some estimates suggest that by 2050 there will be more plastic in the sea than fish!

They say a picture is worth a thousand words. At the end of this chapter I'd like you to stop what you are doing and Google "Plastic - Midway Island." It's really quite shocking to see where some of our garbage ends up. The key to solving this problem isn't recycling. If we all just bought less stuff, we could automatically recycle less stuff.

If you really do have disposable income, think about buying an experience rather than a thing. My wife likes Chris Stapleton (a musician, I think) and has just ordered a ticket to see him perform live. The ticket was more than she wanted to pay, but we justified it because she isn't a typical consumer. Had she paid that much for a new hat we might not have seen eye to eye. My point is this: enjoyable experiences are what tightly bond people together, these lasting memories will be around long after material things hit the garbage can.

It's really clear that the most precious resource we all have is time.
– Steve Jobs

Given half the chance, kids seem to get this concept too. It's funny how they always remember the days when we stopped to color with them on the rug, but quickly forget all the money we spend on plastic toys.

Sometimes we are forced to buy things: roofs leak, cars break, kitchens cupboards wear out. I get it. Reducing stress by reducing clutter is one thing, but the day an unexpected repair bill comes our way the whole stress cycle starts all over again. Don't underestimate stress, it can be a killer, anything you can do to reduce it should be tried. If you are faced with a bill that's over $500 it makes good sense to always get three estimates.

IMPULSE BUYS

Impulse buys on the other hand are a totally different animal. An impulse buy is anything that winds up on your credit card that wasn't a burning desire to buy twelve hours earlier. I'm not sure who wakes up in the middle of the night and says, "Hey, I must buy another windmill for my garden." It's an impulse buy packaged as a bargain along with a gazillion other bits of plastic that we don't need.

For those who need it, the definition of a bargain is something you don't need at a price you find hard to resist.

It's estimated that a single plastic bottle can take 450 years to completely degrade. Perhaps when man has exhausted the world's oil supply it will no longer be economically viable to sail a boat full of plastic goods from China all the way to the U.S. with the intention of then selling those goods on the open market for one dollar each. Given the amount of pollution we are now creating for our children's children, is it me or is it a tad selfish to keep buying more stuff?

Buying less $1 clutter inevitably means less plastic heading for the oceans and landfills. If you aren't sure whether something is clutter or not, try to think of it this way: if you don't love it or use it then technically it's become clutter. The two exceptions to this rule are dangly wind chimes and dreamcatchers, even if you love them they are still clutter, - just sayin.

Tip – for no-nonsense practical advice on how to quit the rat race and live frugally check out a book by the name of Possum Living, How to Live Well Without a Job and with (Almost) No Money, by Dolly Freed.

Sadly, the ones who sometimes seem to get sucked into buying those strategically placed "point-of-sale" items are the ones who can least afford to buy them. Bad spending habits are really just that, a habit that stifles cash flow and increases acidic stress.

One way to break free is to make a list of all the essential things you need BEFORE you go to the store and then stick to it.

THREE STEPS TO FREEDOM

If you need help to peel out of a repetitive cycle of buy, buy, and bust here's an easy three-step way to do it. Step 1: Streamline. Step 2: Use the N-word. Step 3: Repeat.

Step-1: Streamline.

Look around your house and work out which things you absolutely need and what is clutter. How do you know what's clutter and what's not? Simple, if you don't use it, or absolutely love it then technically it's not serving a purpose and it's become clutter. (Yup, worth repeating.)

If at any point you feel motivated to liberate yourself of clutter –don't wait to sell it. Simply drop it off at your favorite charity shop today. Procrastination is the thief of all time.

Step-2 Use the N-word.

This is a little trickier because it takes a certain level of practice to say the N-word right. Stay with me on this, it's a great technique and I guarantee it works. Okay, make an nnnn sound with your tongue (you may need to practice this several times until you feel comfortable.) Only when you have the nnnn sound down can you move onto the next step which is the ohhh sound. Keep alternating between the two sounds and then speeding up until finally a whole new sound evolves.

If you keep practicing the nnnn-ohhh sound over and over it will eventually become shorter. If you are unfamiliar with this sound, it's the opposite of the Yes word. Whenever you go on a shopping field trip make this new sound whenever you see the words 50% discount, final reduction, or half off. Instead of saying Yes, just say Nnnnohhh, (or just NO for short).

STEP 3: Repeat.

From today on, continue using the N-word (NO) rather than hitting the Sales or the Buy Now button. This new sound can help save your sanity, the planet, and your wallet!

Finally, I once heard of woman who was so addicted to shopping that she chose to marry for money rather than love as a way to fund her habit.

At some point in the marriage her purse, containing all her credit cards, was stolen. For two months, her wealthy husband did not to report the theft to the police. When his wife demanded to know the reason for the delay, he calmly explained that the thief was spending less than she was!

What did we learn from this chapter?

Ownership is an illusion; we might think we own something, but if that purchase requires any form of maintenance then it can just as easily own us. Clutter can create self-inflicted stress; the wider implication becomes industrialized pollution.

Homework: please check out "Plastic -Midway Island" a simple Google search should take you there, or click link below

https://www.youtube.com/watch?v=yCb8UKuTzZ0

Chapter 7

SIX TYPES OF DIETS

Over the course of this book dietary information has been slowly bleeding its way through and already we know about toxic food ingredients, excessive sugars, processed foods, deceptive sales tactics, where to buy food, food types, and trigger foods. We've also learned that it can be an incredibly ignorant assumption to think we can lump all our nutritional needs into one single diet. Phew, we really covered some ground today!

So the aim of this chapter is to now guide you toward six diets with a proven track record for success. Some of them you may already know, some you may not. If you are drawn to any one of these diets, great, run with it for a month to see how you feel. If not, no pressure, just continue reading, your answer is in here somewhere – we just have to find it. This isn't a rule book, it's a book to help you find your best fit. And, rest assured, by the time we finish very few stones will be left unturned. So here we go, ready?

It often seems that diet is easily the most divided and confusing topic of all, at times experts will line up to disagree with each other, and finding that single perfect diet can be an elusive dream to chase. A good rule of thumb is don't worry what everyone else is doing, if you find a diet that makes you feel good then keep doing it, if not, consider trying something new. It's safe to say whatever works for the gut flora of one person will not work for everybody. The idea here is to give you several effective options to choose from rather giving you a rigid diet to follow. In the long run, having an open mind will serve you better than becoming entrenched in dietary battle grounds.

Identifying with diets such as raw, vegan, vegetarian, ketogenic, paleo, etc. are great if they are working for you, but don't shoot yourself in the foot over it. The only thing we can say with some degree of certainty is if something comes in a box, a can, or a packet then it needs to be viewed with an element of caution. (I might have mentioned this before.) Before we get too far into this chapter, let's quickly recap.

Often a food product label can be part of a slick marketing campaign and not an accurate reflection of how the food was produced. That cozy "all natural" farm design logo on the label is purely meant to entice you into a making a purchase. Once we become drawn in, food manufactures are keen for us to count units of energy rather than looking deeper at their nutritional content. While calorie counting sounds good in theory, this is a classic bait-and-switch routine that rarely works in practice.

Either way, whatever types of food we perceive to be healthy we then pay for, bring home, and begin spoon-feeding into our bodies. At this point it's important to realize that every time we eat, we are taking something from the outside world and forcing it deep inside our delicate digestive system. I know, right? It all starts with putting the right foods inside our shopping carts.

Avoiding processed foods should be a given, but in today's world, unless a diet has a name to it then it's not really a thing. We could call this the BCP avoidance diet (Box-Can-Packet), some people call it the paleo diet, others lean more toward a ketogenic diet. However, the more mainstream diets become, the more we see it backsliding into foods that are once again trapped inside a box, a can, or a packet. Wherever there is a fast buck to be made, problems inevitably follow.

I've touched on the paleo diet in previous chapters. If you are unfamiliar with the paleo diet then the good news is you can eat as much as you like, you just can't eat everything that you like. For that reason, the paleo diet is a good stepping stone for anyone trying to escape a poor diet because there are no calories to count.

While paleo has obvious benefits, it's worth noting that the standard version doesn't take into account many of the food triggers we mentioned earlier. Fortunately, this time around we are now delving a little deeper and looking to offer you practical solutions. For anyone with a steadfast desire to overcome illness, one of these six classic diets will prove helpful.

1. THE CAVEMAN DIET

Looking at the image below, it seems we are now beginning to evolve into a less than healthy species. Some people refer to the paleo diet as the caveman diet because this is how our ancestors were thought to have fed themselves long before supermarkets came along and made us lazy. Historically speaking, eating fruit when it's out of season or eating carbs out of a box would have been impossible back then, so there are times when claiming to be truly "paleo" can be a bit of a stretch.

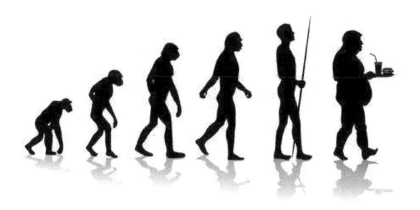

Compared to eating heavily processed foods, a strict paleo diet has obvious benefits – clean, whole foods beat anything you can get out of a can. That being said, we should also exercise a degree of common sense because there are some modern day paleo meals that may have an unnaturally high sugar content. As with any growing trend, everything you could ever need to know is already in print, which is why I'm surface skimming through these diets as opposed to writing a whole book on any one subject. This is good news because finding paleo cooking ideas is now the easy part.

If you are looking for more in-depth answers you can't go too far wrong with the book The Paleo Approach by Sarah D. Ballantyne Ph.D. It's pretty detailed and has a lot of solid scientific background information that's well presented. The author also links to lots of recipes that can be found on her website (PaleoMom) which helps give a clear idea of what the paleo diet is and is not. Again, my role isn't to copy what someone else is already doing right, it's to guide you to good people. For anyone with a suspected autoimmune condition The Paleo Approach is an important book to have on your shelf.

2. THE ELIMINATION DIET

Let's assume that you are already onboard with the idea that the road to health is to eat only whole foods – problem over, right? Meh, not so fast, remember, once you have a spooked immune system all bets are off and you could potentially react to any food, even those found in an organic vegetable grower's garden!

As the name suggests, the elimination diet looks to eliminate problem foods. For anyone just starting off, it is again worth noting that the foods most likely to cause a reaction are gluten, dairy, eggs, and nuts, closely followed by corn. Today, it's not uncommon to find all of these foods on one plate – think of a BLT with mayo. If you can get away with it, great, if not once we simplify the diet anything that causes a reaction is going to be easier to spot.

Ever wonder why you can't eat one cookie or cheese chip? Both gluten and dairy have an addictive quality to them, no seriously, they contain "opioid peptides." Yup, that's the same family as opium. Peptides from both gluten and casein (a protein molecule found in dairy) react with opiate receptors in the brain. Yup, that's right, it has the same effect as if you were taking opiate-like drugs such as heroin or morphine.

When a person comes off gluten and casein they can expect to experience withdrawal symptoms. This is why the cardboard diet described in Chapter 14 is so important – it removes all temptation. (In case you've forgotten, that's the one where you stand before your pantry and refrigerator and toss everything you now know you should not eat into cardboard boxes.) I can't imagine there are too many people who quit smoking or drinking by having cigarettes and booze within easy reach – the same applies to gluten and dairy.

The trick here is to stack the odds in your favor by eliminating suspect foods for a minimum of one month and then slowly reintroduce them into your diet, one at a time. If your symptoms spring back, then bingo, you nailed your kryptonite. To help you do this I recommend picking up a day planner and making a note of everything that passes your lips while making a side note of how you feel throughout the day.

If you (or someone in your family) are reacting to food then keeping a detailed food journal is invaluable because so many foods today have random "things" added to them, things you wouldn't expect unless you were keeping a record. Again keep in mind that in some people reactions can happen much later, hence keeping a written account is very helpful to glance back at. Once food has become a trigger, simplifying your diet will help highlight problems. If this is a new concept to you, then the elimination diet should be something to consider. This isn't a diet to lose weight, it's a diet to lose symptoms. As the name suggests, this involves cutting out certain foods. I get it, changing old habits isn't always easy, but if you are grounded in illness then it's possible that your current diet is either making you sick or keeping you sick. Whenever food enters the digestive system it's scanned for foreign invaders by the immune system. Once a problem is spotted, a code-red is sent out and a reaction occurs, this could result in a food sensitivity or even full blown allergy.

The elimination diet works, yes, and it takes effort, but the rewards for doing it are real. Before we look at the list of foods you may need to break from, let's first take a look at the looong list of symptoms you could be leaving behind. Sometimes we have to give up what we have to get what we want. When you commit to doing the elimination diet you could potentially be saying goodbye to:

- Chronic fatigue
- Arthritis
- Asthma
- Mood disorders, including depression and anxiety
- Skin flare-ups like eczema, hives, and acne
- Autoimmune disorders
- Atherosclerosis (hardening of the arteries, a precursor to heart disease)
- Cognitive decline and neurodegenerative diseases, including Parkinson's and dementia
- Learning disabilities like ADHD
- Trouble sleeping or insomnia
- Muscle and joint pain, such as from arthritis

- Weight gain and obesity
- Migraine headaches
- Nutrient deficiencies
- Kidney and gallbladder problems

The whole point of doing this diet is to pinpoint exactly which foods you are reactive to. You can't always exercise or medicate your way out of a reactive diet. The elimination diet needs to be followed for a minimum of thirty days. When you look at the list of symptoms above, thirty days really isn't that long. This isn't a diet you can throw yourself into half-heartedly, and if you aren't mentally prepared to give it 100% then there is no point in doing it.

Why?

As discussed previously, when the body reacts negatively to trigger foods the immune system makes antibodies to fight the perceived threat. It takes a while for these antibodies to calm down and some believe this process can take three weeks or more. For every cheating nibble you sneak, a new bunch of antibodies are launched and the whole cycle starts over again. Yup, you can hide under the stairs eating trigger foods if you like, but once your immune system is on red alert it never stops watching what you do. For that reason, keep in mind if you cheat you won't feel any benefit of doing the elimination diet and sneaking trigger foods will undermine the whole process.

Before looking at the list of foods you need to eliminate, you might want to make a mental note about why you are doing this. This is a good time to ask yourself WHY you want to be free of your symptoms. For encouragement, take a look at the list above again. And, as you read the list below, note that it is a much shorter list than the list of symptoms you stand to lose. Okay, here we go, take a deep breath, it's time to rip the band aid off and remember that quitting these foods could set you free from a lot of those symptoms in that much longer list.

- No gluten (or any type of other grain)
- No diary
- No soy
- No refined/added sugar
- No peanuts
- No corn
- No alcohol
- No eggs

That wasn't too bad was it? It should come as no surprise that gluten tops the list and, as previously mentioned, you simply can't use this as an excuse to munch your way through the gluten-free section of the supermarket. I never said this was easy but I am telling you it's going to be worth it.

To help you pull this off, check out Tom Malterre. Tom comes to this subject first as a dedicated father of five and, just for good measure, he holds a bachelor's and master's degree in nutrition. His book, The Elimination Diet, is essential reading and is full of tips to set you on the right road, you can also find his talks on YouTube.

3. THE AIP DIET

AIP diet stands for Autoimmune-Paleo and it's a leaner version of the basic paleo diet. It also involves the elimination of all the usual suspects such as grains, dairy, eggs, seeds, legumes, as well as some foods found in the nightshade family which would obviously include tomatoes, tomatillos, eggplant, potatoes, goji berries, tobacco, and all types of peppers. The AIP diet is not without merit as it goes a step further and also removes certain trigger foods such as lectins.

To better understand this diet, your lifeline comes in the form of a well-written blog by the name of autoimmune-paleo.com. The blog is run by two extremely knowledgeable ladies, Angie and Mickey. Both have a well-balanced common sense approach. Their blog is packed with reliable information that is also easy to follow. For anyone struggling with trigger foods, the importance of this information cannot be overstated.

4. THE KETOGENIC DIET

The ketogenic diet is rapidly gaining mainstream momentum. The problem is there is a right way and a wrong way to tap into this highly effective diet. It's fair to say that the ketogenic diet requires an element of self-discipline, but once you get there, food becomes a matter of choice rather a carbohydrate eating emergency. I've been in true ketosis and I liked how it felt, although that's not what I'm doing at the moment. Ketosis also helps clear the mind. But what is this diet and how do we get there?

Think of the body as dual fuel burner, pretty much in the same way a hybrid car is capable of running on either gas or electricity. The body can run on either glucose or fat. At times when glucose is low, the body is perfectly capable of switching fuels. It was once thought that the body only burned glucose for fuel, but we now know that's not strictly true. This is good to know for reasons we will go into later.

Regardless of whether we find ourselves in times of feast or famine, the brain requires an enormous amount of energy to function. When glucose supplies are exhausted, the body begins to convert fat in the liver into energy cells known as ketones. Any time the body burns fat, the metabolic state is described as ketosis. This simply means your body has switched from burning glucose for energy to burning fat. The body has a two-day supply of glucose in the form of glycogen, so the effects of ketosis aren't always immediate. Most people go into a state of ketosis after several days of consuming no more than 20 grams of carbohydrates per day. While this might sound daunting to some, it's worth noting that this is a totally natural process that helped your early ancestors evolve. Back then, food wasn't guaranteed three times a day or any day. Chugging down a quart of orange juice and eating a box full of carbohydrates would have been enough to get you stoned as a witch. Hmm, I see.

The full name of what we are describing here is lipolysis/ketosis. Lipolysis simply means that your fat stores are being burned as the primary source of fuel. The by-products of burning fat are ketones, so ketosis is a secondary process of lipolysis.

Some people refer to this as Ketogenic or Keto diet which is really a just shortening of the term. The ketogenic diet has been around since in the 1920s and was originally started at the John Hopkins Center Medical Center. A ketogenic diet is similar to the paleo diet – however it's typically lower in carbohydrates and high in healthy fats. As always, the devil is in the details because not all fats are the same; some trans-fats can be darn right dangerous! Don't panic, trans-fat (and good fat) is explained in more detail later.

Once the body enters a state of ketosis it becomes more efficient at burning stored fat. For some people, ketosis reduces blood sugar and insulin levels. Some studies also report a marked improvement in diseases such as Alzheimer's, epilepsy, and diabetes.

There are always going to be exceptions, but for me personally, I've found that when I'm periodically in a state of ketosis my thoughts are clearer and I have noticeably fewer food cravings. Essentially what's happening here is we are switching from being a sugar burning mammal into a fat burning one – and some would say this was once our preferred state.

There are a couple of variations on the ketogenic diet which include:

- A standard ketogenic diet which is typically a very low-carb, moderate-protein, and high-fat diet that contains 75% fat, 20% protein, and only 5% carbs.
- A cyclical ketogenic diet which involves periods of higher-carb intake, such as 5 ketogenic days followed by 2 high-carb days.
- A high-protein ketogenic diet which is similar to a standard ketogenic diet, but includes more protein with a ratio of 60% fat, 35% protein, and 5% carbs.

If all that sounds too confusing, then I have the perfect guru for you. Her name is Leanne Vogel and she has a free blog that I urge you to take a look at. Her blog is called "Healthful Pursuit" and Leanne also has a new book, The Keto Diet, that I've just started reading.

As we have already mentioned, ketosis is a normal metabolic process. Unfortunately, its name is sometimes confused with a life threatening illness known as ketoacidosis, an illness driven by a lack of insulin in the body typically seen in diabetics. Although ketosis and ketoacidosis sound alike, they are as similar as chalk and cheese.

It could be argued that ketoacidosis is aggravated as a result of consuming excessive amounts of sugar-spiking carbohydrates. As I'm sure many of you already know, diabetics produce either too little insulin, or the body doesn't respond to insulin at all. When that happens, blood sugar levels can rise and the blood can become dangerously acidic.

Given that the ketogenic diet strives to lower blood sugar levels, it may be something that some type 2 diabetics find useful. As always, before attempting anything new it's best to work it out with an informed healthcare provider.

Although the brain is made mostly of fat, it cannot use fat directly for energy. It can, however, use ketones which the body makes when there is not enough insulin in the blood. From time to time you may hear the argument that the brain needs glucose to run – and while this may be true, it's actually a very small amount. Interestingly, this small requirement can be achieved without resorting to eating donuts. How so? Your body can make small amounts of glucose through a process called gluconeogenesis.

As a final note of caution, keep in mind that although most people do absolutely fine with the ketogenic diet, a sudden switch to consuming 70% fats may, for some people, be too much, too quick. As always, listen to your body for clues which could include pain in the mid- to upper-right section of your abdomen, an indication that stress is being placed on the gallbladder.

5. THE GAPS DIET

Okay, almost there. Four diets down and just two to go. Again, keep in mind that I'm not trying to bust your balls here, I'm simply saying that statistically speaking, there is a pretty good chance one of these diets may benefit to you, especially if your health problems have been difficult to figure out.

At the beginning of this chapter I emphasized that you need to be patient and find the right diet for your unique circumstances. The GAPS diet is another well thought-out diet and some people claim to have success treating autism, ADHD, dyslexia, dyspraxia, depression, and even schizophrenia with this diet.

The only reason the GAPS diet is being mentioned here is because of the dedication of Dr. Natasha Campbell-McBride. I have listened to this lady at length and she has a proven track record for bringing solid results to the table. It also helps that Dr. Natasha Campbell-McBride is incredibly smart and has not one but two postgraduate degrees: a master of medical sciences in neurology and a master of medical sciences in human nutrition.

The GAPS diet has too many benefits to list here, so the list below is just a small cross section of the many advantages people often report.

- Psychological improvements
- Boost immunity
- Reduce food sensitivity
- Improve neurological function
- Heal inflammatory bowel disease
- Improve type II diabetes
- Improve lactose digestion
- Kill candida
- Support detoxification

Dr. Natasha Campbell-McBride is well known for developing a concept known as GAPS (Gut and Psychology Syndrome), which is described in her deeply informative book, Gut and Psychology Syndrome.

6. FODMAPS DIET

Our final diet in this chapter is the FODMAP diet. If you have tried cutting out gluten and failed to see positive results, then FODMAPs are something to be aware of. These are yet another collection of misunderstood foods that can have a foot in more than one category. Just as some people are sensitive to gluten, a person with a FODMAP sensitivity will react in much the same way. For some, FODMAPs are the cause of a wide range of digestive upsets that are particularly prevalent in IBS (Irritable Bowel Syndrome), Crohn's disease, Celiac disease, and just about any other type of digestive disorder you can think of.

What foods are FODMAPs found in?

Many of these foods can be thought of as healthy in their own right which makes awareness all the more important. FODMAPs can be found in a wide range of foods with some foods having a higher count than others. While the list below of FODMAPs is extensive, don't lose heart because there is some good news. This condition is unlike a true food allergy and may even be reversible. A reaction to FODMAPs can be greatly reduced by restricting all FODMAPs for a given period of time to allow the gut to calm down. Are you catching this? I'm saying with a bit of luck; you may be able to slowly reintroduce many of these foods into the diet without too much problem.

Again the idea here is to give you something to grab onto when all else has failed, this time your go-to-gurus are Doctor Sue Shepherd and Doctor Peter Gibson. They recently coauthored a nicely presented book that is actually sitting here at my elbow as I write.

Again as with anyone I choose to recommend, I have no direct link with them other than I admire the good work they do. Doctors Shepherd and Gibson take all the guesswork out of what to eat and what not to eat and it's all neatly covered in their easy to follow book aptly named, The Complete Low FODMAP Diet: A Revolutionary Plan for Managing IBS and Other Digestive Disorders.

In case you were wondering, FODMAPs stands for: fermentable oligosaccharides, disaccharides, monosaccharides, and polyols. If it's easier, we can simply think of them as fermentable carbohydrates. FODMAPS are poorly absorbed by the small intestine and as a result can enter the colon where they are fermented by bacteria, and as they do so, they draw on water and expand causing excessive bloating and diarrhea.

TEST

There is a standard test that your doctor can carry out that doesn't even require blood to be drawn. It's called the Hydrogen Breath Test and it could save you an awful lot of guesswork. Again, rather than let this section overwhelm you, if you have been dealing with stomach issues this is all good information to know. Try to hold onto the positives. You now have a whole list of good people and some new ideas to try and you probably also know a lot more than you did just a few hours ago.

Below is a list of vegetables that are low in FODMAPs, again, let's not forget that some of these foods may have a foot on more than one camp.

Low in FODMAPS = bell peppers, bok choy, carrots, eggplant, common cabbage, endive, fennel, green beans, kale, lettuce, spinach, potatoes, and zucchinis. Fruit low in FODMAPs include bananas, grapes, kiwi, cranberries, lemons, mandarin oranges, blueberries, cantaloupe, honeydew melon, oranges, pineapples, raspberries, strawberries, and tomatoes.

Examples of vegetables high in FODMAPs are garlic, onions, celery, broccoli, all kinds of potatoes including sweet, turnips, sugar snap peas, seaweed, artichokes, asparagus, bean sprouts, Brussels sprouts, and cauliflower. Fruits high in FODMAPs include apple, apricot, avocado, blackberry, canned fruit, cherries, cranberry, dates, grapefruit, mango, nectarine, papaya, peach, pear, persimmon, plantain, plum, prunes, and watermelon.

I get it, some parts of this chapter may have seemed a little heavy, but don't let any of this overwhelm you. The idea is to find what works for you, in order to do this, you have to be aware of your options. Only then can you find the best fit for you. I know you can do this or you wouldn't still be reading. The good news is that more solutions are coming, just hang in there for me.

Life's battles don't always go to the stronger or faster man.
But sooner or later, the man who wins is the man who thinks he can.
– Vince Lombardi Jr

Before we leave this chapter here's a few more foods that are high in FODMAPs.

Grains – wheat and all gluten-containing grains, amaranth, barley, buckwheat, corn, millet, oats, quinoa, rice, rye, spelt, teff, and wild rice

Legumes – cannellini beans, chickpeas/garbanzos, fava beans, kidney beans, navy/white beans, pinto beans, soybeans, peas

Dairy Products – all dairy (except pure butter without additives)

Proteins/Meats – bacon with sugar or maple syrup, broth made with onions or garlic, deli/processed meats

Nuts – cashews, chia seeds, flaxseed, hazelnuts, pistachios

Fats – margarine, soybean oil

Sweeteners – honey, maple syrup, molasses, sugar alcohols, stevia, sucralose, sugar/sucrose

OK, if you made it to this point and you still aren't sure what to do then simply start by cutting out all gluten and dairy for one month. Done right this alone can have a dramatic effect on your overall health, but remember, no cheating. Once you have gluten and dairy under your belt then be sure to try any one of the diets mentioned in this chapter.

What did we learn from this chapter?

Because there are so many variables, some people may have better success with one diet over another. This does not mean the diets recommended here can't work for you, it simply means your individual dietary needs are uniquely different from those of others. A little trial and error should set you on the right track.

Homework: for anyone who appreciates independent values, you might find a TED Talk by Sharyl Attkisson interesting – it's called "AstroTurf and Manipulation of Media Messages."

https://www.youtube.com/watch?v=-bYAQ-ZZtEU

Chapter 8

FAKE-BOOK

As many of us already know, stress is the body's way of flooding the system with hormones in response to any perceived or real threat. Great if there is a Bengal tiger loose in your back garden, but it's not so helpful if you are delayed in traffic and your boss is a jerk.

Stress hormones include adrenaline and cortisol which pump through the body in preparation for emergency action. The good news is short term exposure to stress has no lasting effects. However, a constant level of stress can take a more serious toll on our mental and physical wellbeing.

Medium term stress can manifest itself as headaches, muscle tension, fatigue, stomach upsets, loss of libido, sleep problems, increased levels of anxiety, restlessness, irritability, and sadness. A feeling of being overwhelmed by stress can even change a person's mental state often resulting in emotional outbursts. If stress is left unchecked, a person can easily become withdrawn and depressed.

Have I got your attention yet?

No?

Okay, let's keep going. In addition to the many mental and physical health problems stress can create or exacerbate, it also speeds up the aging process and makes your body more acidic (hello again pH). A constant high level of stress has the potential to disrupt nearly every system in the body! As stress levels increase, immune function decreases, blood pressure rises, and the digestive, reproductive, and nervous systems all get out of balance. Are you getting this? Stress is a killer!

Any sharp increase in blood pressure can result in chest pains, a hardening of the arteries, heart disease, and even stroke, yada, yada, yada. Rather than try to resolve this mountain of health issues, maybe our time would be better spent reducing the main causes of our stress. In part, this can be accomplished when we make more efficient use of our time and take a different view of our spending habits, no really, the time has come to reexamine our reasons for doing what we do, here we go, ready?

MAN-STRESS

Science has shown that men and women react differently to stress. Men have the capability to overreact to overwhelming stress in more extreme ways. I am statistically drawn to the fact that men are three times more likely to commit suicide than women. When stress gets to this heartbreaking level, I suspect it's not one thing that pushes good men over the edge, but a relentless chain of smaller things that have been allowed to build up over time. It's sometimes said that people who commit suicide aren't always looking to end their lives; they are simply looking for a way to end their suffering. If this is you, know that suicide is an irreversible and permanent solution to a temporary problem, if that last sentence didn't quite sink in, I would strongly urge you to read it over again.

Some men find it harder to talk openly to their peers about financial difficulties for fear of being judged. Men may also have a tendency to internalize things far more than women who (generally speaking) often have a better support network of friends in place. Outside of the complications of interpersonal relationships (yup, that would be a whole other book) men generally blame their stress levels on two things: a need for more money or a need for more time – and it's not uncommon for both to be spent unwisely.

Maybe what men are really saying is they would like to be shown more respect. All too often men are encouraged to relate success with owning objects, hence men feel the need to make more money which in turn requires more time. It really doesn't help that men are constantly bombarded with idiotic statements from luxury brands like car manufacturers like Porsche who claim that "there is no substitute" for owning a $250,000 car. *Really?* I've driven a Porsche and it really didn't bring me any peace.

Let's not forget that men are also frequently targeted by expensive diamond retailers who are keen to tell you, "Diamonds are a girl's best friend." If men only knew, ownership is an expensive illusion and inner peace doesn't come from what we buy; it comes from the things we can live without. If you can't freely give away what you own, then you don't own it, it owns you.

While we all have different income streams, each and every one of us gets the same amount of allotted time every day. What we spend our time doing is a choice. Some men may spend it chasing the latest car, a new suit, a bigger desk, all of which are rewards for having too much money. But these are short term rewards that cannot compete with having the freedom to do what you want when you want.

> A man is a success if he gets up in the morning and gets to bed at night, and in between he does what he wants to do.
> – Bob Dylan

So what's the solution for a chronically stressed man who has fallen into the trap of equating success with ownership of more stuff? That's easy – remember 102-year-old Edie Simms from chapter 8? Turns out she was right; you can actually liberate and sooth your soul by simply humbling it. *Are you getting this? It's kinda important.*

Edie does something on a regular basis that not only keeps her going, it's been scientifically proven that her life is enriched every time she helps another person. No really, there is enough scientific data about that to fill the rest of this book. The term "Helper's-High" is based on national research done by Allan Luks (feel free to Google) which revealed the powerful physical feelings people experience when directly helping others— results were measurable and showed improvement in both physical and emotional health.

Friend, it's not your money I'm after; it's you. Time has a value; the love of money gets people into this mess. The fastest way to alleviate any type of self-inflicted stress is to find a problem that's bigger than you are. People are hurting all around you, and yet there is something uniquely valuable about looking another person in the eye and saying, "Hey, are you okay in there, Bud?"

In today's fast-paced world we have become quick to measure ourselves by the quality of the car we drive, the size of our houses, or the number of electronic digits we have that represent our net worth. Perhaps a man would be better judged not by economic wealth but by the way he treats the most vulnerable members of a society.

Trust me when I say this, to someone who's going through hell, the simplest of human interactions can be more valuable than the shiniest of gold. Look at it this way, every year, one million of the world's poorest people die from drinking contaminated water. When you stop and think about it, that's a heck of a lot of people with a very basic need that is not being met.

On the flip side, eight men now control as much wealth as the world's poorest 3.6 billion people. According to a new report from Oxfam international, Bill Gates, Warren Buffett, Carlos Slim, Jeff Bezos, Mark Zuckerberg, Amancio Ortega, Larry Ellison, and Michael Bloomberg are collectively worth an eye-watering $426 billion. Don't get me wrong here, it's their money, they earned it and good luck to them. But to have an abundance of money parked in a bank, would suggest there is a little wiggle room in the budget to help the little guy find water, am I right? Okay, where am I heading with this? Why do we suddenly expect the superrich to step in and help, when we are not prepared to give a little of ourselves? Lord knows, it's not difficult to find worthy causes.

Look, I know for some, this may be stepping out of your comfort zone but the fastest way to finding your own sanity is to help another person. No really, I can back it up with actual scientific studies later, but for now, I'm offering you a way out of this shitty cycle, take it!

> Man is not made for defeat.
> – Ernest Hemingway

The trick here is to do a little but do it often. This doesn't have to be a huge drain on your time. Maybe offer to help a sick or elderly neighbor, at the same time try to be respectful of the fact that the transition into vulnerability isn't always and easy one.

I get it, committing huge portions of your time can lead to frustration. The idea here is to do what you are comfortable with rather than turning it into a form of resentment. For this tip to work it doesn't matter how little you do, so long as you do something. What do you have to lose? If I'm right, you will begin to get back something your money cannot buy – a quiet sense of inner peace. No really, have you ever wondered why volunteers don't ask for money? It's not because they have no value, it's because they are priceless!

Your inner peace is out there waiting for you. You may find it helping out at a local soup kitchen, or you may find it volunteering at a local hospital; you know your personality better than I do, find something you are comfortable with. Do this and a month from now I swear you will be happier and less stressed, you'll also care less about your neighbor's stuff. If anything, your neighbor will be looking over YOUR fence thinking, hey, what's with this guy and his new inner peace?

Do this quietly and for the right reasons. Work for a cause, not applause. There's no point if this morphs into a boasting opportunity and no, you don't need to tell the world via a Facebook post what you just did for someone. If you think men have it bad, try walking a mile in a woman's shoes - don't get too excited, I didn't mean that literally.

WOMAN-STRESS

Women have an added stress. Almost every woman who engages with any type of media is immediately faced with images of younger women with increasingly bigger eyes, bigger lips, bigger boobs, and even bigger butts. Sheesh, way to make a person feel uncomfortable in her own skin. If that isn't stressful, I'm not sure what is.

Today, one of the primary causes of stress for women is the constant pressure to conform to a certain physical type in order to be accepted. Social media has become quick to present us with a carefully staged digital image of perfection, but scratch below the surface and you sometimes find the deep roots of insecurity. Perhaps the world doesn't need more skinny women taking selfies in bathroom mirrors. It needs more normal, content looking people doing stuff your grandma used to do. I sometimes wonder if it's called a "selfie" because narcissistic is too difficult a word to spell? I digress.

More than ever, people are desperate to show you an updated snapshot of their happiness, often this is nothing more than an elaborate hoax in need of debunking. When your Facebook feed is constantly bombarded with photos of people having 24/7 fun, it's important to understand that not everything is how it seems.

Example: I once watched a young mom take at least ten grinning selfies next to a shimmering hotel swimming pool, and yet standing off to one side was her small child in a damp polka dot bikini complaining that she was cold and hungry. Given the time it took the woman to get the perfect selfie I have probable cause to believe the kid with the tears in her eyes failed to make it to the final cut. Maybe a better name for Facebook would be to call it Fake-book. I guess one advantage of not having a Facebook profile is you don't have to worry whether people "like" you or not ... just sayin.

At times, social media can be a warped distortion of reality where nothing much is the way it seems. It can even make us feel as if we aren't enough. Recently I read an article about how some women in the U.S. are so desperate to fit in they turned to an illegal underground practice where bigger butts are offered on the cheap. Sadly, this is done by injecting dangerous chemicals under the skin. These butt-boosting shots include injecting mineral oil and a can of roadside tire inflator directly into the muscle. Nope, not joking.
If you haven't seen this product before, it's sold in car accessory shops and its intended use is to inflate a blown tire with rapid set expanding foam. I know, right? What kind of message is social media sending out to impressionable young minds when it makes them feel as if they need to pump it up with fix-a-flat tire weld?

Perhaps our wives, sisters, and daughters are constantly being told that in order to fit in they need to have a totally different body shape. Might I remind those who are caught in this trap to look at any old photo of a family member to see how quickly ridiculous fashions come and go. Once it might have been a curly perm, tall platform shoes, or a pair of flared jeans. Bad fashion is one thing, but can you imagine ten years from now looking at a body that has been surgically altered to meet a current fashion trend?

It would seem that even the clothing industry is geared to keep young women hooked on buying more clothes. Given that the global apparel market is currently valued at an eye-watering three trillion dollars, fashions now change before you can say the word overdraft, often leaving some women feeling compelled to buy a new outfit every day of the week!

Trying to extract value from ever-changing fashion is just another form of negative stress and, left to ferment, it simply becomes unhealthy.

> Buy less, choose well.
> – Vivienne Westwood

I get it, we all long to be accepted, but in the process our minds have become polluted with an unsustainable lust for material things. I say to you, reading this right now, take comfort from the fact that your uniqueness has value – it sets you apart from the crowd, so FCUK the fashion industry, dare to be different!

So, just as men are striving for more respect from their peers, it seems women, above all else, just want to be valued, but that value needs to come from within. Regrettably, wants and needs are two very different things.

For sure, we all need clean food and water, a warm safe place to sleep, and clean clothes to wear. We all want a friend to turn to in our time of need – but beyond that, it rarely bodes well to have an emotional attachment to material things. Believe me, I appreciate that letting go of such things ca be a challenge. It might surprise you to know, as I write this I'm currently in the middle of giving up my home, here's why.

HAPPY HOMESTEAD

For the past ten years, home has been set in the Northern mountains of New Hampshire. It's not a big place or a fancy place, but my wife and I had made memories here. Over the years we had worked to transform this property into a super-efficient homestead. With a small flock of chickens and several sheep, this little gem became the absolute epitome of sustainable, simplistic living and minimalism.

After overcoming my earlier illness, the word "home" took on a whole new meaning. This place had since became an integral part of our lives, it gave us clean food and safe shelter from the outside world; it's been our school, office, church, and hospital. Flanked on all sides by organic gardens and fruit trees, it's fair to say that every inch of this land had been worked and it had just begun to give back more than it took. Over in the barn, my small collection of hand tools could all be found neatly lined up on the work bench like a surgeon's operating table. We were intentional about living this way, growing our own food was important to us, in short, we bothered no one and no one bothered us. Here's where it gets tricky.

Make no mistake growing food is hard work, to help me do this year round I built a small high tunnel to extend the growing season. This final addition was an important piece of the puzzle because it allowed me to grow clean food through the winter. Little did I know at the time, but this "improvement" was going to be my downfall.

Unfortunately, I must have built it a little too well because it quickly provoked a visit from the town tax inspector who was sniffing around for a reason to increase my property taxes. I guess he liked what he saw because over the next twenty-four months our property taxes steadily increased by several thousand dollars. When you just want to live a simple life, this rate of increase was not only unwelcome it was, sadly, unsustainable.

If I'm honest I'm still a little irritated by this. Ultimately we were being priced out of the small town we had come to love. But with no sign of the man letting up, we calculated that our property taxes had almost doubled. Given the history of the two countries, you know somethings not right when an Englishman gets to complain about American taxation.

Rather than watch our property taxes go up again, we decided to put the place up for sale, this had become a matter of principle as well as economic hardship. As I'm still in the middle of writing this book, perhaps later we will see if this if this was a mistake or not. Either way, a lady from Florida saw the photos online and was immediately smitten. She flew up the very next day and said it was the sharpest looking house she had viewed to date.

She particularly liked the warm, friendly feeling of our home and kindly commented on how clean everything was. Her husband was suitably impressed with the efficiency of this house which could be heated year-round with just four cords of wood.

This was really important to him (just as it had been to us) because he wanted a small place with affordable utility bills. It seemed to tick all the right boxes, but after several days of deliberating, the wife finally decided not to buy. The reason?

She had once travelled to Japan and while there had bought a large collection of ornamental china vases that she then imported to the U.S. For the past fifteen years, wherever she lived, they lived. No matter how hard she tried in her mind, she simply couldn't find a place in our house to put them all. As her husband rolled his eyes for the third time it made me realize this was a classic case of something they no longer owned. These vases truly owned them!

The love of possessions is a weakness to be overcome.
– Alexander Eastman

Long story short, someone else soon came along and snapped it up. This actually brought heaviness to my soul, but it also made me thankful that we had owned this house and all of its things, while none of them owned me.

For now, this American dream has come to an end and we have decided to sell everything we own and try our luck back in the motherland. As liberating as this may sound, it's probably the first time I've packed a suitcase and not wanted to be somewhere else.

I'm really not sure where the wind will take us next, and although we will miss the stability of our home, my message to you is clear: things shouldn't define who we are, because one day, things may come or they may go. When all else fails we must simply dust ourselves off and keep going.

Finally, I'd like to ask you for just four minutes of your time and direct you to an unusually short but inspiring four-minute TED Talk. Mark Bezos is a volunteer firefighter and he quickly retells a short story of heroism that didn't quite go as expected — it taught him a BIG lesson which was don't wait. You can find him in today's homework section below. Enjoy!

What did we learn from this chapter?

Stress can also come from having too little money while trying to own too many things. It can also come from the media, and yes, even social media. We can quickly reduce our stress levels by finding a problem that's bigger than we are, more on this coming.

Stress can also make us more acidic, a subject we seem to keep coming back to. We can reduce our own stress levels by finding a cause bigger than we are.

Homework: Make time to watch this four-minute TED talk by Mark Bezos, this guy is my kind of hero!

https://www.ted.com/talks/mark_bezos_a_life_lesson_from_a_volunteer_firefighter

Chapter 9

THE WEAKEST LINK

Take a sneaky look behind any website and you will see long lines of computer code. Take a peek behind the dashboard of your car and you will find lots of wires. Take a hard look at the underlying cause of illness and you will almost certainly find that its roots are deeply intertwined with chronic inflammation. Wait a second are you catching this? There is a link between serious illness and inflammation!

Inflammation is associated with just about every health condition; even PubMed is awash with strong scientific data connecting inflammation to a list of diseases ranging from cancer to obesity. Given the importance of this, perhaps we have things a little twisted. In every hospital we have swarms of oncologists, cardiologists, and neurologists, *but not a single inflammation-ologist!*

We have a medical system that's rich in cash and yet fails to address the underlying cause of chronic inflammation. During a routine doctor's visit it's not unusual to hear your doctor talk about preventative medicine and yet the root causes of inflammation are rarely mentioned.

What's interesting is that developing countries that spend statistically far less on healthcare consistently outperform the West on everything from infant mortality to longevity. *I know, right? What's up with that?*

Allow me to repeat myself with emphasis: inflammation and illness go hand in hand. Given the importance of this subject, let's take a look at what inflammation is and then see how all this fits in with what we have learned so far. Inflammation is an essential part of the repair process within the body; it can be acute or chronic. Many of us will have already experienced acute inflammation which is an early-stage response to obvious physical trauma (think of a twisted ankle or bruise). Acute inflammation is obvious and rapid. It will include an onset of pain, heat, redness, and swelling. This is also a sign of a body that's healing. Think of acute inflammation as being similar to a small campfire that's under control.

Chronic inflammation, on the other hand, is less obvious and has more of an insidious quality to it that can span weeks, months, or even years. As the diagram below suggests, chronic inflammation is the common denominator that's weaving its way throughout so much serious illness. The good news is that chronic inflammation is totally reversible. If this is true, it suggests that many illnesses are also reversible – but you already know this because of course you watched the suggested homework video in Chapter 5.

Think of chronic inflammation as a smoldering, lingering type of fire always on the lookout for a puff of wind. Once chronic inflammation ignites, it can be likened to a raging forest fire.

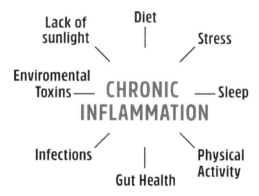

Looking at the diagram above, can you see how all this is beginning to fit neatly together? If illness has you in its grip, there is a pretty good chance that something in this image led to your downfall. And by the same token, something here also holds the key to your recovery!

These eight categories can be thought of as our pillars of good health. The good news is once we get these bad boys in line, good health is yours for the taking!

We seem to have covered a lot of ground together and I fully appreciate it can be a lot to take in. The idea of this chapter is to take stock of what we have learned so far. Just to keep things interesting I'll be mixing in a few new things that I hope you will find interesting. If repetition is the mother of all learning, let's quickly begin our short recap with stress and continue working our way around the diagram in a clockwise fashion.

STRESS

In this life there is no shortage for the causes of stress, some of these we have already taken a look at. Stress has become an omnipresent part of life and even with the best intentions it can follow us around like a bad smell. The people we surround ourselves with can bring us stress and certainly our jobs can.

Everything of true value either has a heartbeat or it is free. With that in mind, the one category we do have full control over is the things we buy. As discussed previously, our value should not come from material things nor can it be found in the approval of others.

I will not let anyone walk through my mind with their dirty feet.
– Mahatma Gandhi

Magnesium plays an important role in stress reduction. Long- to medium-term stress will quickly deplete magnesium levels. Certain foods such as dark leafy greens, avocados, and almonds have a high magnesium content. Do a little homework and you will find there are others.

Stress can also lower the function of the immune system making us more susceptible to infections. One way to combat stress is to increase the things in your life that bring you pleasure. It's very hard to remain stressed when you are doing something that gives you joy. If eating junk food gives you pleasure, then sorry, you can't include that. Nice try though.

SLEEP

Although we should aim for a minimum of six hours, some people will absolutely need more. The quality of our sleep is just as important as the quantity. Sleep is where our body gets to work cleaning the brain and accomplishing all those internal repairs; sleep is like the maintenance crew that comes in to do essential shop cleaning at night. For this reason, it's important to protect your sleep. Keep your bedroom cool, dark, and quiet. Avoid all forms of blue light in the evening because it will disrupt melatonin production.

Around bedtime be mindful of what you eat. Sugar and protein will almost certainly keep you awake; instead, go for clean carbs at supper such as a bowl of rice. We aren't trying to win culinary awards here; we are looking for a better night's sleep. Medications and certain health supplements can also disrupt our sleep. If you are having trouble sleeping, try not to take anything after 6 p.m. You can find more sleep tips in Chapter 24.

PHYSICAL ACTIVITY

Cells like movement and all motion is lotion for the joints. As discussed earlier, even something as simple as bouncing on a small yoga trampoline can have a big impact on our health. These types of trampolines are relatively inexpensive and allow the user to ease into exercise at their own pace. Personally, I like the trampolines sold with springs and the one I have is called "ANCHEER." For some people, joining a gym is never going to happen – that's okay. If committing to an exercise program is a step too far, look for cheats like parking your car farther away from the store. This becomes a subtle way of forcing us to walk. A brisk walking is less traumatic on the body than running long marathons. Whenever we exercise, our lungs begin pumping more oxygen and this helps with the pH of the body. Remember, sitting is the new smoking!

Incorporating a hobby makes exercise less of a chore which means you are more likely to do it.

Prior to selling my tiny homestead, I managed to get my daily workout from gardening. This usually involved a lot of bending and lifting. Providing you don't overdo it, lifting is an important part of any exercise routine because it helps maintain testosterone levels. Contrary to what you may think, women also produce testosterone, albeit in much smaller quantities. Low testosterone can cause symptoms ranging from low sex drive to depression.

GUT HEALTH

This is huge in more ways than one. We might think of the skin as being the largest surface area to come into contact with the outside world, but some estimates suggest that if the GI tract were laid out on the floor it would fill a tennis court! The gut is the cornerstone of your physical and mental wellness. Repairing the diet doesn't happen overnight, foods loaded with excessive sugars are intended to be addictive and it takes effort to change. Gluten and dairy also have an addictive quality to them which is why it's so difficult to "just have one." Poor diet and medication can fuel the destruction of those delicate gut bacteria.

Sometimes we have to make a leap of faith so I need you to just trust me when I say your mental state is often a reflection of your gut bacteria. Feeling grouchy all the time has more to do with your gut than your brain. The good news is this is fixable.

Some medications prescribed to alleviate symptoms can have an adverse reaction on gut bacteria. As we've discussed, antibiotics can be lifesaving but indiscriminate overuse of antibiotics has become a huge problem coupled with the fact that antibiotics are now regularly used in the food supply. Restoring gut flora takes time; treat it as a steady marathon and not a sprint. Fermented foods and probiotics can help, but it's best to do this slowly. Keep in mind we don't want to cause the bad bacteria to die off too quickly or we will feel worse. Some people are drawn to yogurt for their probiotic content. Be aware that store-bought yogurt is often pasteurized and is more likely to be filled with sugar than any useful probiotics.

Food plays a key role in both gut health and inflammation. Years of eating the wrong foods cannot be overturned in a day. Be patient, the road to recovery takes time. Foods that heal rarely come from a tin, nor do they have a high sugar content. Bone broths are covered in more detail later and they are a valuable tool for anyone looking to repair the gut.

INFECTIONS

Infections can be caused by living organisms such as fungi and bacteria. Some of these organisms cause disease while others can be quite harmless and some even help our bodies work properly, including those found in the gut. Trillions of these bacteria and other microbes are already living inside your body and it's often said the number of microbes inside us outnumber our cells by about ten to one! Essentially we are a collection of bacteria with a human host. I know, right? Who are we, really?

Bacterial, viral, fungal, and even parasitic infections all receive their nourishment from you. Often in illness we alternate between hot and cold sweats. In the short term this can be a positive sign of healing. A fever is a common sign of illness, but that's not necessarily a bad thing. In fact, fevers seem to play a key role in fighting infections as some illness-reducing pathogens are killed off at higher temperatures.

Understanding that fevers play a key role in fighting infections means you will need to exercise a degree of common sense when deciding whether to let a fever run or call the doctor. As a rule of thumb, if you are an otherwise healthy adult, not immunocompromised or taking chemotherapy drugs, and haven't recently had surgery, then up to 102 F (38.9 C) it can be beneficial to let a fever run – but, obviously, drink plenty of fluids to stay hydrated. Ultimately this is dependent on your circumstances. It's not a hard and fast rule and it's not intended to replace medical advice.

Most common infections are no match for an immune system that's supported by good nutrition. The problem is we don't always realize this until after we become sick. Antibiotics are sometimes used to treat certain infections. While they obviously have a place in medicine, overuse brings its own problems and antibiotics won't do anything to treat any type of viral infection.

Natural alternatives worthy of further investigation are tea tree oil, colloidal silver, cistus-incanus tea, food-grade-hydrogen peroxide, and MMS 1. The latter two being the most controversial, but they are both treatments I have used in the past to good effect. Am I saying they are right for you?

No, I'm saying here are five separate things that are worth more research. In the right diluted dose, some things are helpful and others can be darn right dangerous! Dose is the key to EVERYTHING, even common table salt when eaten in too great a quantity is deadly. Heed the warning: moderation will always serve you better than excess.

ENVIRONMENTAL TOXINS

Industry is fueled not by oil, but by consumer demand. It's estimated that by 2050 there will be more plastic in the sea than fish. These tiny plastic partials are now entering the food chain and nobody knows the long-term effects of this. The most effective way to recycle is not to buy it in the first place. Buying plastic goods in ignorance is no longer sustainable or acceptable. THE MOST EFFECTIVE WAY TO DEAL WITH PLASTIC ISN'T TO PUT IT IN THE RECYCLE BIN, IT'S TO STOP BUYING IT!

SUNLIGHT

The positive effects of broad spectrum light on the body are wide reaching and profound. Think of a summer evening around 7 p.m. – most main streets are a hive of activity as people walk around feeling alert and awake. Natural sunlight plays a key role in how we feel. Natural light also affects mitochondrial function – these are the tiny energy cells of the body. Now think of a dark winter's night around the same time. By 7 p.m. on a winter's night some of us are probably already in our PJs, right? Light is energy, embrace it!

Sensible daily exposure to sunlight also helps our bodies produce vitamin D which is essential for healthy immune function. Sunlight also increases dopamine release in your body. Even plants grow measurably stronger when exposed to sunlight.

DIET

Food has a profound effect on our health and yet today food is such a loosely defined term. Clean, locally grown food often has a higher nutritional content than large scale commercially farmed crops. When you buy local it's a WIN-WIN – your community thrives and you get to eat food that's in season and at the peak of nutritional value. As a commodity, food is often exploited; as a medicine, food is often misunderstood.

Typically, fast food also has excessive amounts of manmade sugars. This will drag the immune system down and deplete the body of key minerals. All food turns to sugar anyway, and dumping more into the system only adds to the problem. Fruit is naturally high in sugar. In nature we wouldn't find everything ripe at the same time or in the same place. Fruit was meant to be eaten in moderation and in season. Until you get your health issues under control, consider giving fruit the boot. You can slowly reintroduce it into your diet later. When the body can no longer cope with the amount of sugar circulating in the bloodstream, the problem goes well beyond diabetes. One illness loves sugar above all others and its name is cancer.

Today most fast foods are cooked in vegetable oils which have been shown to cause oxidative stress; this simply means the oils create free radicals in the body which in turn causes inflammation. Oils high in omega-6 will promote inflammation, as will dairy products and grains. If this is all new to you, don't panic.

If you are new to the subject of nutrition and feeling overwhelmed by it all, a good rule of thumb is to simply fill half of every plate you serve yourself with organic leafy vegetables. Do this one thing and your portion sizes will naturally become more balanced and tackling the remaining 50% of your plate will be less daunting.

KIDNEY, LUNGS, SKIN, and LIVER

Treating symptoms is as easy as popping a pill but unless the underlying cause is addressed, progress will always be slow. When we become ill our delicate filtering organs such as the kidneys, lungs, skin, and liver are already working under pressure. Everything we swallow has to be processed, so let's be aware of the things we ingest whether they be food, liquid, or pills. In effect, the things we swallow can tax the body; this is even true of vitamins and herbal supplements (as previously discussed).

A healthy liver is essential to good health because it does far more than just detoxify toxins. If one organ above all others deserves the title of being a true multitasker, then it's the liver. It performs over 500 different functions, including fighting off infection, neutralizing toxins, manufacturing proteins and hormones, controlling blood sugar, and helping clot the blood which is probably the reason for it being the largest and heaviest of all the internal organs.

The liver is the most metabolically complex organ in the human body. It plays such an important role that it's the only visceral organ to possess the remarkable capacity to regenerate itself. Get this: if part of the liver is surgically removed or chemically damaged it can actually regrow itself. I know, right? It has to be the coolest tool in the toolbox and any time you are ill you can bet the liver is either being overused or abused.

A liver that's been overworked can sometimes outwardly manifest as frustration or increased emotional instability. If you find yourself easily crying, becoming easily irritated, or acting out in anger, look to the liver. To help improve liver detoxification naturally, a castor oil pack is sometimes used. The idea is to apply a liberal amount of high quality castor oil to a piece of cloth, then place it over the liver and hold in place with a hot water bottle to help stimulate lymph and liver function. A simple Google search will give you the exact details for this effective protocol. Another way to assist the liver is to drink fresh lemon juice first thing in the morning (see Chapter 15).

It seems highly probable that if we have a problem with the liver we can also expect underperforming kidneys because the two are so closely intertwined. Once the liver and kidneys are struggling to cope with the demands put on them, you may also notice an increase in body odor. When the kidneys are underperforming, itchy skin conditions such as eczema may also flare up and odor is prominently noticed in the feet.

Another reason for increased body odor (and there are many others) could be a low-grade biofilm infection. Cistus-incanus tea is something worthy of further investigation. When used over a two-week period, most infections give up and the body odor disappears. As always, moderation will serve you better than excess, and small amounts of tea taken regularly is more helpful than excess.

Gentle herbs such as milk thistle can be helpful to detoxify the liver. Herbs have been used safely for thousands of years, but as with anything that detoxifies – go slow or risk dumping toxins into the bloodstream faster than they can be removed. Using herbs that support the liver and kidneys may help bring an improvement to overall health.

Enlisting the help of a knowledgeable, local herbalist can bring faster, safer results. Be mindful that the effects of other drugs/supplements can be magnified as they are dragged through the liver or kidneys. Where possible, it's best not to mix/take them at the same time.

Sodium bicarbonate has been shown to be helpful with certain kidney issues. You can find this in most regular supermarkets and it's often called baking soda. The preferred brand is sold by Arm and Hammer because it doesn't have any other ingredient apart from sodium bicarbonate. It's important that it has NO aluminum added as with some other brands.

Before you rush to shoot me down for suggesting you drink baking soda, let me first tell you that this research comes direct from the Royal London Hospital and findings can also be found published in the Journal of the American Society of Nephrology.

As always, do your own research and before trying anything new always speak to your doctor. I sometimes find it helpful to add a quarter of a teaspoon of sodium bicarbonate to a glass of water and drink it on an empty stomach.

Another firm indicator that the kidneys are running out of sync is a change in urinary frequency, either too few trips to the bathroom or too many. These are often reflected in the color of the urine, i.e., too dark or too light. This was already covered in some detail at the end of Chapter 7.

Let's not forget that the skin and lungs form part of the detoxification process. Problems with the lungs are obviously easier to notice because anything that affects breathing is instantly going to be on your radar. Here, the herb mullein can be an effective ally along with staying hydrated.

Mullein helps lubricate the lungs and throat membranes while reducing swelling, which can help alleviate irritation. Mullein has traditionally been used to remedy bronchitis, asthma, croup, whooping cough, pneumonia, asthma, and tuberculosis. It can be made from loose tea and sipped, or in tincture form added to water. As always, my goal is only to guide you to these things and your role is to research them to the point where you make your own judgment calls. Keep in mind these are delicate filtering organs; less will always serve you better than more.

I've long suspected that people with a passion for a project usually hang around long enough to see it completed. In my honest opinion, this is one of the more powerful tips offered in this book which is why I'll be covering it again in another chapter. Having a purpose (in spite of an illness) can get us through the toughest of mental days.

Look, I know it sucks being ill and, trust me, you can go back to being ill for the rest of the day, so for now just humor me. Find something – anything – that is important to you, even if it's only for five minutes a day. Make no mistake, a passion, when combined with a determined spirit, is a powerful tool to have in the box. People who are passionate about finishing a project rarely seem to die while in the process.

There is no right or wrong answer here. You can commit to painting a landscape or a bedroom at your own pace. Fly a kite or fly a plane, make a video or write a book, start a club or join one, plant a tree or cut one down – it's all good.

Even if I knew that tomorrow the world would go to pieces;
I would still plant my apple tree.
– Martin Luther

What did we learn from this chapter?

Illness is always going to go after your weakest link. It's well documented that chronic inflammation is behind a wide range of diseases. The good news is it is reversible. This means that something in this chapter could be your silver bullet.

Homework: for a better understanding of how things link together in the body, check out "How the Body Works," by Dr. John Bergman.

You can find this video on YouTube. Over the years I've gotten a lot of solid information from this person. Or click the link below:

https://www.youtube.com/watch?v=mActHjsX5pc

Chapter 10

MY DIET IS BIGGER THAN YOUR DIET

Ask ten foodies what constitutes a healthy diet and you are in for a polarized debate. It seems no topic is more divided than what should go on the end of your fork. Making a claim to be vegan, paleo, vegetarian, a raw foodist, or ketogenic has almost become like pledging an allegiance to a particular religion. And once the rigid battle lines are drawn, people are quick to become defensive.

Vegans and vegetarians – know that I feel your pain and much of the advice, information, and suggestions in this book should guide people away from barbaric farming practices. But at this stage, encouraging someone who is just now seriously thinking about nutrition to go 100% vegan is simply a bridge too far. Raw foodies – know that I have no beef with you either (yup, intended pun) and we could endlessly debate the pros and cons of yours and other diets, but the most important and first thing I want to stress is that any dietary choices that take us away from the heavily processed and very sad SAD (Standard American Diet) are important steps in the right direction.

Rather than divide ourselves into opposing groups, can we at least all agree that if your diet makes you feel great then it's the right one for you. By contrast, we can say with equal conviction that if you are experiencing a number of health issues perhaps your diet has room for improvement. When our thinking is rigid it's easy to prove ourselves right, but in the process we run the risk of shooting ourselves in the foot.

Let's also remind ourselves that so much of this is open to interpretation. A person eating pizza, fries, and cake could technically claim to be vegetarian, just as a person eating deep fried chicken and fries could claim to be paleo, and someone on the ketogenic diet could certainly be eating greater than normal quantities of cheese. Are these healthy, balanced ways to eat? I would say not. However, the idea behind this chapter isn't to tell you what foods to eat, it's to look at your current diet with a view to plugging any nutritional gaps it might have.

Everything I have learned (and continue to learn) has come as a direct result of trying to keep an open mind. Periodically, I find it helps to write down everything I know about nutrition on a blackboard and then wipe the blackboard clean. Looking at problems from different perspectives allows us to see things we might have missed. Who knows, perhaps nutrition started to go wrong as far back as Columbus when he decided to inflict his discovery of potatoes, corn, and tobacco on the rest of the world ... *just sayin'.*

MITOCHONDRIA

Mitochondria are a fascinating subject and what you are about to read is an oversimplification of probably the most amazing and powerful sequence of events your body performs every second of every day. While simplification helps us cover more ground together, I have to say that the subject of mitochondria warrants a book solely devoted to it. This, clearly, is not that book.

But fortunately, there are two new books on this very subject. The first is Dave Asprey's book Headstrong. Dave did a real nice job on this and for sure it's worth checking out. Not to be outdone, Dr. Joseph Mercola has just released a new book titled Fat for Fuel. As with anything Dr. Mercola puts out, it's a wealth of cutting-edge information.

Mitochondria are tiny cigar-shaped batteries found inside almost every cell in the body. They can be thought like the battery in your car. When that battery is fully charged, the engine bursts into life on demand, but when the life of that battery is almost drained your car's engine is slow to turn over.

When mitochondria perform well we feel energized and healthy. Mitochondria really don't care what particular diet group you belong to; they simply demand raw materials to make energy. You can take it to the bank that when the mitochondria are undernourished, illness, fatigue, and brain fog are all present. Let's take a closer look at nutrition from the mitochondria point of view.

Mitochondria are perfectly formed powerhouses that produce energy by utilizing oxygen and breaking down food and then releasing that energy in the form of ATP (adenosine triphosphate), along with some byproducts such as carbon dioxide, water, and free radicals. ATP is the fuel of the cell and it's used for everything from blinking to sprinting. Why is this important?

Think of it this way: we can go months without food, we can go days without water, we can go minutes without air, but when it comes to going without ATP? Meh, you have about fifteen seconds before it's game over. ATP is the energy currency of life and it's mostly produced inside the mitochondria. We could think of ATP as gasoline used by a car, but as we all know, gasoline doesn't come straight from the ground ready to use, it has to be refined from oil.

Making ATP is a process similar to refining oil and it happens mostly inside the mitochondria. Given that we cannot go fifteen seconds without making ATP, we could argue that this process is more important than the air we breathe. Can you see where I am going with this?

We know that the highest numbers of mitochondria can be found in the brain, eyes, and heart, and in women there are also high concentrations of mitochondria in the ovaries. Rather than asking which set of dietary rules we must defend and obey, let's flip the question around and ask, hey, what do my mitochondria need to function optimally?

When we look at nutrition from this perspective we will do well to remember that the greatest number of mitochondria live in the brain – and as we already know, the brain has an extremely high fat content so it makes sense that we need to consume foods that are high in fat. Duh. This doesn't mean we have to throw all other diets under the bus, it simply means we should increase the fat content of the foods we choose to consume.

This also highlights the problem of following a strictly low fat diet which, as it turns out, makes absolutely no sense whatsoever. I know, right? WTF? (Where's-the-Fat?)

Fat goes by lots of different names, including saturated, unsaturated, polyunsaturated, healthy, unhealthy, trans-fats, omega-3 fats, omega-6 fats, etc. This is a topic fraught with confusion and, depending on who you ask, everyone seems to have a different opinion.

GOOD FATS

While it might not be politically correct, I'd like to simplify this mess by splitting it into only two groups: good fat and bad fat. Be warned, in some circles even these can be viewed as the same thing – remember, mitochondria really don't care what advice others have for you, they just need the raw materials to function optimally. One of those raw materials is good fat. Not all fats, however, are equal.

Let's first look at fats found in animal products like grass-fed butter, whole raw milk, and fatty meats. I don't expect everyone to agree, but in my opinion these are all good fats. Butter sometimes gets a bad rap, but the devil is always in the details. Cows that graze on open pastures make the best butter and it's nothing like the margarine humans make. You know that, right? Manmade = bad.

Other sources of good fats can be found in avocados, pasture-raised eggs, coconut MCT oil, raw cacao butter, and raw nuts such as pecans and macadamias. These types of fats are friends to your brain.

Animal fats contain beneficial levels of (good) omega-3s. Omega-3s can be found in healthy fish such as Alaskan salmon, sardines, and anchovies because these fish are lower in toxins. Krill oil supplements can also help boost omega-3 and they generally have fewer problems than regular fish oil supplements because they have a lower mercury content.

Omega-3 fatty acids are a class of essential fatty acids. The two principal omega-3 fatty acids are EPA (eicosapentaenoic acid) and DHA (docosahexaenoic acid). For all ages, DHA is critical for optimal brain function. If you want your kiddo to be smart, best you pay attention.

Omega-3 is essential for optimal brain health and, in a perfect world, omega-3s should be balanced with omega-6s. A balanced ratio would be in the approximate range of 1:1.

Unfortunately, the standard western diet has this balance massively out of whack in favor of omega-6s. Some estimates put this imbalance as high as 25:1 in favor of omega-6! When the ratio of omega-3 and omega-6 is out of balance, the stage is set for inflammatory health problems. As mentioned earlier, inflammation is heavily implicated in all forms of illness. Hmm, I see.

High concentrations of omega-6 fatty acids can be found in vegetable oils – for example, per tablespoon grape seed oil has as much as 9744 mg; sunflower oil, 9198 mg; corn oil, 7452 mg; wheat germ oil, 7672 mg; soybean oil, 7059 mg; shortening, 4771 mg; and margarine, 3323 mg. With so much of fast food being fried in these types of oils, it's easy to see why the balance is so far off.

BAD

The real kicker is that foods high in good fats are sometimes shunned by the medical profession. For this we can thank a flawed study by the late Dr. Ancel Keys. His work linked higher saturated fat intake to higher rates of heart disease and ever since it has stuck in the minds of some doctors. But the problem isn't healthy fats – it's another group of fats known as trans fats. Trans fats can really mess with your insulin receptors. Some research suggests that trans fats can even increase your risk for chronic diseases such as cancer, heart disease, and diabetes.

Personally, I try to steer well clear of all commercially fried foods because they tend to be fried in trans fats. Trans fats are found in margarine, vegetable shortening, and partially hydrogenated vegetable oils. Trans fats are just unhealthy and you should avoid them entirely – they are typically used in low-quality products and your mitochondria can't use them (so neither can you). Trans fat = bad.

Bad fats aren't helpful to you or to your mitochondria; it's the equivalent of trying to build a house with substandard materials. As we seem to have come full circle back to talking about the nutritional needs of your mitochondria, let's also kick out all those excess sugars, processed flours, gluten, and dairy. Ahh, that feels better already.

Avoiding trans fats, as well as taking gluten and dairy off the table, is a good starting point. Do you remember why? The correct answer is gluten and dairy (closely followed by eggs and nuts) have the highest probability of triggering an unwanted food reaction. As a gentle reminder, let's keep in mind that gluten isn't only found in bread, it's in pastas, pastries, crackers, cakes, cereal, granola, pancakes, waffles, croutons, sauces and gravies, flour tortillas, brewer's yeast, and just about anything else that has wheat flour as an ingredient.

When you have an immune system that's watching everything you do, you can't cheat even a little. To keep things interesting, it gets even trickier when eating out because it's in soooo many other foods.

I suspect Mitochondria also enjoy an abundance of fresh vegetables with a wide variety of colorful greens. Ideally aim for six to nine cups a day. Sulfur rich foods can help the body produce glutathione which you can find these in cruciferous veggies: bok choy, broccoli, cabbage, cauliflower, horseradish, kale, kohlrabi, mustard leaves, radish, turnips, and watercress.

There is some debate surrounding the goitrogenic effect of some of these foods which are thought to affect thyroid function by inhibiting synthesis of thyroid hormones. While this may be true in extremely large doses, cooking and steaming reduces this effect. So, too, does supplementation with selenium, vitamin E, and iodine – but let's not get ahead of ourselves when there are still plenty of food options on the table.

Without wanting to veer too far off topic, it's worth repeating that taking either selenium or iodine in isolation has the potential to causes more problems than it solves. This synergistic gang of three should be taken in direct relationship to each other. Other supplements that can be thought of as mitochondria-protectives include acetyl-l-carnitine, alpha-lipoic acid, coenzyme Q10, N-acetylcysteine, NADH, D-ribose, resveratrol, and magnesium aspartate. But for now, let's stick with food.

Fiber is important for good digestion and can be found in fruits, vegetables, and grains. But because we are trying to avoid grains, here's a list of foods that are high in fiber but do not contain any grains: avocados, Asian pears, berries, coconuts, figs, artichokes, peas, okra, acorn squash, Brussels sprouts, turnips, black beans, chickpeas, lima beans, split peas, lentils, nuts, flaxseeds, and chia seeds. Seeds and beans are best soaked overnight to aid digestion. Men and women have slightly different fiber needs. It's recommended that women get approximately 25 grams of fiber a day and men between 35 and 40 grams.

Autoimmune conditions can wreak havoc on the mitochondria. If you aren't sure whether or not you have an unrecognized autoimmune condition remember that a good indicator that you do is if you've seen multiple doctors and are still without a firm diagnosis. The joy of autoimmunity keeps on coming and anyone with this condition should also consider the possibility of a leaky gut. If this is you, then bone broth can be a useful food staple because it is rich in glutamine and other amino acids known to be beneficial for the lining of the gut.

CRUISING FOR OYSTERS WITH JACK

There can't be too many controversial neurosurgeons out there smart enough to make your head hurt and abrupt enough to cause offense. If you are blissfully unaware of Dr. Jack Kruse, be warned – his critics call him an undiplomatic quack and his supporters label him a revolutionary genius.

Personally, I find his style refreshing although his stance on mercury fillings is at odds with my own experience. Dr. Kruse is very aware of the dangers of mercury teeth but has chosen to keep his as removal can be equally dangerous. Perhaps it's the mercury in his own teeth that makes his style somewhat abrasive. Either way, the magnetic pull of Dr. Jack Kruse is something I find strangely fascinating.

You are probably wondering why we are suddenly talking about a controversial neurosurgeon, right? I'm glad you asked. Whether you love or dislike him, there is no getting away from the fact that Dr. Kruse is incredibly smart. It's also fair to say the average brain surgeon knows more about the brain than the rest of us. Dr. Kruse is on the absolute cutting edge of innovative medicine and when he talks, I listen.

Dr. Kruse sometimes catches flack for being too far out there, but he's basically a proponent of eating paleo, keeping seasons in mind, eating more ketogenic in the winter and more carbs in the other seasons – something I think most people can get their heads around.

In his professional capacity, Dr. Kruse is quick to tell us that DHA is an important brain nutrient. He also believes that of any food, oysters are the most nutrient dense for optimal functioning of the human brain. Is he right? Who knows? But whenever I come across fresh oysters I now eat them and so far I've lived to tell the tale.

Oysters have no central nervous system, so the theory is they do not feel pain. Perhaps this might sit well with vegetarians looking for an alternative protein? Oysters are considered a powerful aphrodisiac and a good source of essential minerals including phosphorus, calcium, potassium, and zinc. Some people eat oysters raw and do just fine with them. For my money I prefer to have them cooked because there is a risk of raw oysters carrying the hepatitis A virus. It's really not the oysters' fault; Hep-A is sometimes found in water that has been contaminated by humans.

Cooking oysters is super easy. Simply place the oysters in a flat bottomed pan and add a little water. Slowly apply medium heat until the oyster shell opens and, bingo, you are good to go. The whole process usually takes between five to ten minutes.

The US Food and Drug Administration also warns that oysters should be cooked to avoid contamination with pathogens. And of course, a good rule of thumb is if something doesn't look or smell right, throw it out. My final tip is to only buy oysters if the month has the letter "R" in it. Colder months generally provide a better crop.

What did we learn from this chapter?

While it's true that not everybody is going to have the same dietary needs, we can with absolute certainty say that everybody has mitochondria. When the mitochondria are fired up they go hand in hand with good health. The eyes, heart, and brain all have a high density of mitochondria.

The brain needs fat in the diet to function optimally. The ideal ratio of omega-6 to omega-3 fats is 1:1. You can help maintain this balance by regularly taking krill oil supplements and eating fish such as Alaskan salmon, sardines, and anchovies because these fish are lower in toxins.

Homework: check out Jack Kruse.com.

https://www.jackkruse.com/

Chapter 11

SEVEN BIG GUNS, NO CARROTS

In this chapter we will look at six things that have nothing to do with food but can have a profound effect on your overall health. The good news is each one is easy to do and totally free! Every day I try to incorporate some aspect of these things into my daily routine.

#1 SET THE CLOCK

With the precision of a Swiss clock, birds migrate, flowers open, roosters crow, and at 5:15 p.m. every evening it was common for two deer to walk through the back of my property. I suspect neither of them owns a wristwatch, and yet they must absolutely have body clocks. Animals, plants, and humans all respond to changes in darkness and light. These changes follow the approximate 24-hour cycle and have a profound effect on physical and mental health. This cycle is better known as the circadian rhythm.

Like the deer, we also have a body clock and there's a price to pay when it's out of whack. Fortunately, resetting it is pretty easy to do. For best results, this should be done each morning within five minutes of waking by simply exposing yourself and your eyes to as much natural sunlight as possible.

If you find yourself stuck indoors on a dull, overcast day, be sure to open the blinds and turn on lots of bright lights. Setting your clock is a two-part trick. To keep your circadian rhythm in check, it's also essential to keep to a regular bedtime schedule. I get it, establishing consistency takes discipline, but I promise you, the rewards for doing this are rapid and real.

Science recognizes that a "master clock" in the brain coordinates all the other body clocks so that they are in synch. Circadian rhythms influence hormone release, body temperature, sleep-wake cycles, and hundreds of other important bodily functions. Abnormal circadian rhythms have also been associated with diabetes, depression, obesity, bipolar disorder, seasonal affective disorder, etc. Sleeping in on weekends can throw your whole body clock off; if you need extra sleep on the weekend, try going to bed earlier. For those of us who are now too old to rock but too young to die, this is easy advice to follow.

The importance of keeping the circadian rhythm in sync cannot be overestimated; a brisk walk in the morning sunlight is an incredibly powerful way to give you an immediate energy boost as well as help you reset your circadian rhythm. When your eyes sense morning light, your body responds by being more awake and alert. For that reason, be sure not to obscure the sunlight with sunglasses. Did I just say you need to stare at the sun until your retinas bleed out? No, of course I did not. That would be idiocy.

As the evening sun sets we want the opposite of bright light. The electric light has been an invaluable asset to mankind, but as the evening rolls in we risk sabotaging not only our circadian rhythm but our melatonin production. Keep in mind that before the invention of the electric light bulb humans relied heavily on the soft glow of candlelight. Today we are bombarded with harsh blue light almost around the clock.

In most houses, electric lights throw off a harsh blue light. This is also true of LED lights and compact fluorescent bulbs. You may recall from an earlier chapter that some of those compact fluorescent bulbs (the curly looking ones) have mercury in them! The best solution is to use a small evening lamp, preferably with one of those older incandescent light bulbs – something with an amber glow will suffice.

Humans are the only species bright enough to make
artificial light and stupid enough to live under it.
– Jack Kruse

Bottom line: after dark it is important not to confuse our brain into thinking it's still daytime. Some of the worst culprits for artificial blue light are laptops, tablets, and cell phones. Be sure to power down tech devices at least three hours before bed. You can also apply a filter to them such as F-lux. This is available as a free download and it works really well.

#2 BEAT-STREET

Check this out: in 1994 the Journal of the American Medical Association (JAMA) published a study showing that surgeons performed measurably better while listening to music. The best results happened when music was selected by the participants. Hmm, I see.

Music can reach into parts of the brain faster than a shot of tequila. A recent study showed that music improved cognitive performance and recall abilities in patients suffering from dementia. Music has also been shown to reach Alzheimer's patients where medications fail. I recently put this to the test when my wife and I went to visit an elderly relative. Serious illness has been ravaging her ailing body for quite some time. She can no longer speak, is bedridden, and spends her days staring at the ceiling. Familiar voices mean nothing to her and are often met with a blank stare. But the day my wife played her favorite hymn, "Amazing Grace," I swear, her eyes opened wide and she turned her head and smiled.

Music has the ability to lift the soul. Sometimes we just have to be reminded to use it as part of our daily health routine. Whenever I find myself in a funk, the fastest way I know of to turn my day around is to jump on a small trampoline while listening to a short music video via YouTube.

They say you can tell a lot about a person from the music they listen to. Personally, I can find something to bob my head along to in just about any music genre. I know, right? Square peg, round hole.

When my body dies, my wife knows to play Louis Armstrong's, "What a Wonderful World" going into the church and, just to keep the energy up on the way out, I've requested "I'm a Firestarter" by the Prodigy (true story). Like me, it seems my musical taste is a little difficult to put into a box.

For just a moment I'd like to challenge you to imagine living in a world with zero music. (I know – bummer.) Now write down three of your favorite songs. At the end of this chapter I'm going to ask you to play them. See how quickly music has the power to stir up your emotions. Obviously you want to steer away from sad songs; the idea here is to lift your spirits.

#3 EARTHING

If I had to choose only one tool to tackle illness, that tool would be an open mind. Opening ourselves up to new ideas allows us to see problems from a different perspective. You might want to hold onto that thought as we now look at grounding, also referred to as earthing.

For consistency, I'll use the latter term from here forward. We like to think we are biological beings but really that's only part of the story. Your brain, heartbeat, and neurotransmitter activity all rely on electrical signals. Without these electrical signals there would be no life. Fundamentally, you and I are electrical beings.

149

To be clear, there are plenty of credible, published scientific studies surrounding earthing. More important, earthing is something you can put to the test for yourself right now and monitor your own results. If the weather outside allows, try reading the rest of this chapter outside with your bare feet touching grass, stone, or concrete. This experiment will not work on asphalt (that's tarmac for my European homies).

I know what you are thinking because I thought it too – what's with this hippy shit, right? Do yourself a huge favor; postpone your judgment until you have all the facts. Better still, ask yourself when the last time you placed your feet on bare earth was. For many of us, this probably happens once a year on vacation. Walking barefoot on the beach felt good, right?

Apart from that beach vacation, the rest of the year we keep our feet wrapped in plastic boxes, walk on nylon carpets, drive our cars on rubber tires, and expose ourselves to ridiculously large amounts of electromagnetic pollution. If I were a gambling man, I'd bet the farm that these events play a huge part in systemic inflammation. Why?

When you look at blood samples under the microscope the differences between earthed and non-earthed blood is quite remarkable. It's sometimes said, what can't speak can't lie. When the two samples are set side by side it's almost like looking at red wine and tomato ketchup. Make no mistake, earthing improves blood viscosity.

It seems the smarter we become, the dumber we become. Maybe future historians will look back on this period the same way we look back on the Roman Empire. Those Romans became so smart they began moving water around in lead pipes which we now know is a toxic heavy metal. It wasn't long after they began doing this that the empire crumbled from within. Perhaps over time Wi-Fi will be the equivalent of lead pipes.

Studies reveal that earthing has an effect on heart rate variability, cortisol dynamics, sleep, autonomic nervous system (ANS) balance, and reduces the effects of stress. In short, earthing helps put out the fire of inflammation! If you take only one thing from this chapter let it be this: earthing is missing in our modern day busy lives, illness is not!

Earthing appears to minimize the consequences of exposure to "dirty electricity." How often should you practice earthing? If you are exposed to Wi-Fi daily, then it pays to make this a daily habit. I try to do this every morning, ideally for twenty minutes a day – longer is better, and less is better than nothing.

Tip - Anytime you find yourself unable to think straight, find a quiet spot outside, slip off your socks, and let your feet touch the negative charge of the earth. This allows the transfer of electrons to your body which in turn helps neutralize damaging free radicals. In a relatively short space of time, the world and all its problems begins to look like a very different place.

Earthing can be done any time simply by making contact with the earth or walking barefoot outside. In parts of the world where walking barefoot isn't possible, there are now special shoes that incorporate copper contacts into the soles. Long before manufactured rubber soles became the norm, leather-soled shoes acted as an effective semiconductor. These types of shoes were sometimes worn by our Victorian ancestors.

Earthing devices are not restricted to shoes. Today it's possible to purchase an earthing mattress, mattress covers, and even pillow cases that work by using the ground plug of a house. Although you tend to get what you pay for, some people report deeper sleep with less mind chatter and fewer aches and pains in the morning. In one study, participants who slept on a special earthing mat showed significant changes in key biomarkers including serum sodium, potassium, magnesium, and iron.

The key to effective grounding indoors is to ensure your outlets are properly grounded because all grounding mats use the ground wire in your home. If you are in any doubt, ask an electrician to check them for you.

Sleeping while earthing makes good sense because you don't have to do anything other than sleep to reap the benefits. For those who are more technically minded, you can see the difference this makes when you hold a simple voltage meter. To better understand what's happening, think of earth as being abundant in negative ions. Another ideal place to have a grounding mat might be at your feet as you work on your computer. If you find yourself on a limited budget, you can make an earthing mat with a few basic supplies from a hardware store. YouTube has lots videos to show you how to do this. Ideally, whenever you use a laptop put it on a desk. If you don't have a desk, try placing a thick book beneath it along with some kind of pillow. This will help reduce the EMF felt in the body to some degree.

If you really want to be blown away by earthing, invest in Clinton Ober's book Earthing: The Most Important Health Discovery Ever? Just reading the reviews on Amazon will make your head spin!

#4 COLD THERMOGENESIS

WARNING: cold thermogenesis may not be suitable for those with a serious health condition, please consult a medical doctor before trying it.

Compared to wandering around shoeless with a flower in your hair, cold thermogenesis is a little more hardcore. While it's not for everyone, if you can pull this off the rewards are plentiful which is why it's a favorite with top sports people to aid in recovery. There's also a couple of easy cheats to help you do this.

Cold thermogenesis helps alleviate pain, improves mood, and increases production of norepinephrine in the brain (which is connected to focus and attention.) It's also known to be helpful in reducing inflammation and can even help with migraines. But wait, there's more. Cold thermogenesis is said to lower body fat, increase sexual performance, and improve adrenal/thyroid function. If it feels like I am giving you all the benefits before revealing exactly what cold thermogenesis is, you are correct. Why?

Cold thermogenesis involves cold water, a bath of sorts, and you. I know, right? Had I opened with that you would have probably stopped reading by now. Fear not, cold thermogenesis was something I stumbled upon even before I knew it had a name. Back in 2011 my body intuitively knew the value of cold thermogenesis and given how ill I was I just went with it. Years later I was surprised to learn there is actually a lot of published scientific data to support this concept.

At the time, my sitting in ice cold water must have made it seem as if I'd lost my marbles. No doubt my wife (bless her) had me pegged as bat-shit crazy, but it's one of the many things I've done that helped in my own recovery. The part that left my wife scratching her head was when I started doing it outside in the dark. Why?

With inflammation raging through my body, the outside temperature had dropped to where I needed it, and doing it in the dark spared the neighbors having to see a sickly looking, semi-naked Englishman sitting outside in a tub of ice cold water. WAIT! Before you turn the page on me, remember I have some cheats to help get you through this. You don't have to do what I did to get a benefit. The good news is you can tap into cold thermogenesis gradually by starting small. There are a couple of ways to do this.

Method #1: for this you need to find a pan the size of your face. Fill a third of it with water and then place the pan in the freezer. Once frozen, take it out and top off the bowl as needed with cold water. Next, place your face in the ice water for as long as you can stand it. The first couple of times you probably won't be able to do it for more than a few seconds but over the week you should be able to withstand it for longer periods. Congrats – you are experiencing the benefits of cold thermogenesis with all your clothes on.

Method #2: you could try incorporating the James Bond shower from an earlier chapter, yup, that old chestnut's back. The easy way to do this is to start by taking a hot shower and then gradually turn the water to warm and then in the last thirty seconds of your shower, on cold. Aiming the cold water on your face and chest may also help you breathe easier throughout the day. The cold water also stimulates the lymphatic system. Gradually, easing into this rather than jumping into a cold shower makes the whole process less daunting, and believe me, once you get used to it, it's actually quite invigorating – *no, seriously.*

Method #3: over time you may feel ready to take the plunge and try an ice cold bath (obviously assuming that your doc says it is okay for you to try). It's easier to do cold baths if you focus on the benefits of doing it and it may help to start off with lukewarm water and gradually add in more cold.

You might not be able to do this for very long to begin with and that's okay. Over time I managed to do it for half an hour at a time without even shivering, although I suspect if I tried it today I'd be lucky to do a few minutes. If you try this, it's helpful to keep your head, fingers, and toes out of the water because these extremities are particularly susceptible to cold. A final word of caution to men: when you get out of a cold bath it's probably not the best time to take that naked selfie ... *just sayin'*.

#5 LET THERE BE LIGHT

Recently, while passing an antique shop, I happened to notice in the window an old light box for sale. The box measured approximately 4ft x 4ft with a hole in the top for a person to poke their head through. Inside, the light box was lined with mirrors and lights. Back in the day, a person would pay to sit inside the box and have their body blasted with light.

What's cool about this box is the company that made it also installed the exact same model on the Titanic. This made me think, light therapy really isn't anything new, but it's incredibly powerful. Here's why.

The skin acts almost like a solar panel charging up the body with ultraviolet B waves and a cholesterol derivative found in the skin. Once the skin comes into contact with natural sunshine (or light that mimics sunshine) vitamin D (which is actually a hormone) is synthesized.

Make no mistake, light has a profound effect on the body and the aim of artificial light therapy is to mimic elements of natural sunlight. Light therapy is known to affect brain chemicals linked to mood and sleep. But wait, there's more.

In 1903 the Nobel Prize for medicine was awarded to Niels Ryberg Finsen for his outstanding contribution to the treatment of diseases, particularly Lupus vulgaris which is a form of tuberculosis (TB). This was treated with concentrated light radiation. Finsen believed that tissues that had been attacked by bacteria might respond well to treatment with light.

In 1895 he used concentrated beams of ultraviolet light to successfully treat patients with lupus vulgaris. For a time, light therapy was widespread but was eventually replaced in medicine with antibiotics.

Today, some smaller light therapy boxes can fit on a desktop and are designed to help those with seasonal affective disorder (SAD). This is a particular type of major depression that occurs at specific times of year when sunshine is least available.

Exposure to a light box for as little as thirty minutes a day can help stimulate a change in the hormones that affect mood. If you live in a part of the world where the sun doesn't shine, then you really should have a light box (otherwise called a SAD lamp) somewhere in your house. You can find light boxes for sale at Amazon.

The benefits of natural sunlight cannot be understated. Any morning when the sun is shining I immediately make a beeline outdoors to get a skin-full, preferably before the geoengineering-gods see fit to block out the blue sky. I know, right? Humans controlling the weather, what could possibly go wrong?

RED LIGHT THERAPY

Red light therapy differs from the light therapy just described. Again, it's light that you can see but, as the name suggests, it's light that comes in the form of a red glow. There are a couple of different types of red light and they each play a different role. In this section you need to pay attention to those differences because understanding them will impact your health in different ways.

Red light therapy falls into the visible light spectrum between 630-700 nm on the electromagnetic scale. Red light therapy is often used to treat the surface of the skin. Red light therapy can be thought of as healing and regenerative; it accelerates wound healing and can be applied to muscles or joints to reduce swelling or pain.

Last year I pulled something in my shoulder while working and I used red light therapy to help fix it. I liked using this option because it's noninvasive and drug free. There are lots of options out there, some offer good value for the money and others can be quite expensive.

The one I've been using lately is made by a company called Tendlite. It's the size of a flashlight but don't let the size fool you. It's really well made and a powerful tool to have in the toolbox for relief of joint pain. Relief doesn't always happen overnight, but if you stick with it results do come.

As with any of the following therapies, it's important to keep the light away from your eyes. Ideally you should invest in a set of inexpensive goggles similar to those used on some tanning beds. The light sold by Tendlite comes with dark glasses.

Tip – If you are on a shoestring budget, simply purchase a red heat bulb found in most pet shops. They are often used to keep young chicks warm and come with an inexpensive lamp holder. Bingo – you have a red light therapy for less than twenty bucks!

Red light therapy also soothes inflamed tissues, is good for headaches, sinus pain, nasal congestion, sore throats, earaches, and coughing. Red light therapy can help you get a deeper, more restful night's sleep, promotes relaxation, and is known to reduce anxiety and irritability.

Okay, now here's where we switch to a totally different type of light so it's important to make the distinction. Before you dismiss this idea you should know that the folks at NASA were early proponents of the following types of light.

INFRARED (AND NEAR INFRARED) THERAPY

Here we are talking about two different lights, the main distinction relates to the wavelengths. Infrared light typically falls into the invisible part of the light spectrum with wavelengths between 700 and 1200 nm, while near-infrared light falls into the spectrum of 700 nm to 2500 nm. Of the two, near-infrared can be thought of as deeper penetrating,

Near-infrared frequency can have a healing effect on our individual cells. Inside the mitochondria of every cell there are receptors that respond to near-infrared wavelengths. This light triggers an increase in cell metabolism, protein synthesis, and antioxidant activity which helps the cells detoxify. Near-infrared light reduces inflammation and pain while simultaneously triggering growth and regeneration in the cells.

Near-Infrared light comes to us in the form of halogen, laser, and LED. The preferred technology is LED because the surface temperature can be controlled. It also disperses over a greater surface area giving a faster treatment time. Near-infrared LED also has a gentler delivery, will not damage tissue, and carries less risk of accidental eye injury.

Benefits of near-infrared therapy are

- Boosts metabolism
- Recharges mitochondria
- Stimulates white blood production
- Reduces body fat
- Promotes cell regeneration
- Increases energy
- Reduces inflammation
- Improves circulation
- Heals wounds faster
- Provides pain relief
- Rejuvenates the skin
- Lessens joint and muscle pain

If you have the means, you can look into investing in your own infrared sauna. For the rest of us, we can tap into this technology by joining a local gym that has an infrared sauna as part of its membership. If you spend enough time researching the health benefits of light, it isn't long before you come across the name of Dr. Joseph Mercola (whom I've mentioned before). Dr. Mercola was talking about light therapy long before it became mainstream.

Dr. Mercola is a highly reliable source for cutting edge medical news and I use his site often. If you are looking to expand your knowledge, I urge you to check out his vast library of videos at mercola.com.

#6 FIND YOUR IKIGAI

This is probably the most important health tip in the whole book and here it is tucked away almost undetected, perhaps one day I'll write another book on this very subject. The Japanese have a word for it: it's called ikigai (pronounced ee-kee-guy). Roughly translated, it means having something to get out of bed for in the morning. It's your reason for being. Make no mistake – having a project you are passionate about can help keep you out of the doctor's office.

Every one of us has something we enjoy doing even if there is no money involved. It's as if the human soul is hardwired to have a purpose. Take my advice, if you want better health, go find your ikigai. When you learn to tap into what motivates you, something happens at the biological level. Ever notice how motivated people rarely get sick?

Lately, this book has become my ikigai and here's something freaky to ponder on. Every day for the past year, I've known deep inside, that there wasn't even the slightest chance that I was going to croak half way through writing this book. Nope, was never going to happen.

Perhaps you have already noticed in your own life how certain projects or times just feel different. A Monday morning feels vastly different than a Saturday morning, am I right? Both days have the same number of hours, so what's changed? As kids, many of us remember that Christmas morning feeling when we bounced out of bed at 5 a.m. Yet trying to get out of bed on a school day always felt like a challenge. Obviously not every day can be Christmas, but it serves to make a poignant point: having a meaning adds purpose to a person's life.

#7 LAUGHTER IS MEDICINE

Finally, it's sometimes said that laughter is the best medicine, unless of course you are laughing out loud for no apparent reason, in which case I suspect you need some medicine. Learning to laugh in the face of adversity is a powerful cure for all known stress. At some point during the day, give yourself permission to smile, even if it's only for a minute.

Sometimes when my wife and I were waiting at the hospital, I'd see a worried look come over her face. The challenge was always to find something to make her laugh so hard that no sound would come out and she would be forced to clap like a demented seal. It really was a beautiful sight.

> A wonderful thing about true laughter is that it
> just destroys any kind of system of dividing people.
> — John Cleese.

What did we learn from this chapter?

Each of the light therapies in this chapter offers a wide range of health benefits. Light therapy can affect mood, circadian rhythm, and many other body processes. Red light therapy is helpful with joint and muscle pain and near-infrared therapy can act as a cell rejuvenator, among other things.

Homework:
- Play your favorite song as loud as you possibly can!
- Check out Dr. Mercola at mercola.com, here's the link.
- https://www.youtube.com/watch?v=1xxP1e4zQ7c

Chapter 12

LIQUID LIFE

Water is water right? Meh, not so fast. Science tells us that water can occur in three phases: liquid, solid, or gas. Liquid water is wet and fluid. Water as a solid is water that freezes. And water as a gas is the vapor present in the air all around us. But what if I told you there was a 4th phase to water that's rarely talked about and yet has a profound effect on your health?

This is not H20 but rather H302 – it's more alkaline, dense, and thicker than regular water, and it's actually alive and even holds a negative charge much in the same way that a battery does. In terms of benefits to you and your health, this living water is capable of tackling a wide range of health problems with astounding results.

When you have this piece of the puzzle in your toolbox it changes everything and, nope, it's not holy water. This 4th phase water is already inside you and by the time this chapter ends you will know how to give it a boost and where to get even more of it. Most medical students learn that water is just a background carrier to more important chemicals and bacteria, but according to Dr. Gerald Pollack, a PhD in biomedical engineering, water is central to everything the body does, and in relation, everything the cell does.

As early as Chapter 5 we first began exploring the idea that a healthy body requires healthy cells and now that concept comes full circle. An average adult is thought to be made up of 50-65% water, with the percentage of water in infants being much higher, typically around 75%. This type of water isn't the same as the water we drink from a plastic bottle. This water becomes highly-organized and appears in abundance inside most of your cells, even our extracellular tissues are filled with it.

Dr. Pollack has published numerous peer-reviewed scientific papers and his understanding of the physics of water is uniquely valuable to anyone in search of better health. Dr. Pollack carried out extensive experiments at the University of Washington on this 4th phase of water which uncovered some remarkable findings. One experiment showed that the water molecules acted like telephones to carry messages throughout the body. Dr. Pollack's team also discovered that this type of water has the ability to exclude things it doesn't like, even small molecules. Given this unique property, it's sometimes referred to as "exclusion zone water" or EZ water for short.

The negative charge found in EZ water helps form cellular energy. Are you getting this? Your body is made up mostly of water and that water is alive and it takes what it needs and excludes what it doesn't. It then sends signals around your body creating enough energy to keep you moving throughout the day!

Light is a key ingredient for creating EZ water, whether in the form of visible light, ultraviolet (UV) wavelengths or infrared wavelengths that we are surrounded by all the time. If the goal is to maintain wellness or recover from a serious illness, it's important to understand that energy comes from the light we absorb which in turn affects the cells.

Laser therapy can help increase EZ water by penetrating the cells. In doing so, some laser therapy treatments have also been shown to reduce pain and inflammation which can help shorten healing time in muscles, ligaments, and bones.

Infrared light is the most powerful, particularly at wavelengths of approximately three micrometers. Hence the reason infrared sauna may prove helpful because the cells in the body are deeply penetrated by infrared energy which in turn helps build EZ water. The same can be said for spending time in the sun, although to get the full benefits of natural sunlight you need to step outside rather than sit behind a glass window. Glass will filter out much of the natural light spectrum. For the same reason, if you are a wearer of glasses you may find it helpful to periodically remove them and let the natural light gently and indirectly filter through to your eyes.

The fear surrounding natural sunshine and skin cancers is not without justification, but it might surprise some to know that statistically speaking skin cancer rates failed to go down when the use of sunblock became more widespread. Equally confusing is the fact that many skin cancers appear on parts of the body the sun doesn't reach.

Sunshine also plays an important role in the way your mitochondria communicate. Increased vitamin D levels play an important role in creating EZ water. Am I saying you should stay in the sun until your eyeballs burn out? Nope, that would be foolish. But keep in mind some of those sun blocking creams contain toxic chemicals, and anything that goes onto the skin goes into the bloodstream. Who knows, perhaps over time some of those toxic chemicals may prove to be equally problematic … just sayin'.

Sun in moderation appears to be the preferable key. Personally, I try to get a skin full of sun in the morning before midday. If the afternoon sun is strong I either stay shaded or cover up with a brimmed hat and long sleeved shirt to give my arms some protection. Let's be clear, full spectrum light from natural sunlight is important to your health, manmade light by comparison can be more of a problem.

Spend enough time under fluorescent tube lighting and some people begin to experience fatigue and even migraine headaches. If you are particularly sensitive, even LED lighting can have a negative effect. Given the number of hours we spend indoors, as mentioned earlier it may be a better option to switch back to the older incandescent type light bulbs (obviously not those curly ones that contain mercury).

Light aside, EZ water can also be found in glacial melt, but unless you have a spare iceberg in the back garden you might want to consider locating a natural deep spring, the deeper the better because EZ water increases when under pressure. There are actually some products on the market that attempt to emulate this natural process by creating something known as vortexed water. Personally I haven't used any of them so I can only speculate about their effectiveness.

Vibration also plays a role in increasing EZ water and, to a lesser degree, so does rebounding on a trampoline. Movement is important to your health. If for some reason you find yourself immobilized with ill health there are products on the market to help achieve the sensation of intense movement. Whole body vibration plates come in all shapes and sizes and can be a useful tool to anyone standing or sitting at a desk for long periods of time.

If you don't have access to a vibration plate, an underground natural spring, an iceberg, natural sunlight, or infrared light, then fear not, all is not lost. EZ water can also be extracted from living foods, which brings us neatly to the subject of juicing. Juicing is simply a way of squeezing the juice out of vegetables and fruits and then drinking the liquid. I know, right? But just trust me on this one. There are few things capable of turbo charging your health faster or better than juicing!

If you are unfamiliar with this term you are in for a pleasant surprise. Juicing can form part of any diet which simply means you can dip your big toe in the water without too much disruption. Done right, this process doesn't just boost your nutrient intake, juicing also helps clean out the GI tract which can over time become clogged with mucus, rancid fats, undigested proteins, and parasites. I know, right? It's nasty, but a cleaner GI tract will result in better absorption of nutrients into the cells.

The idea that you are what you eat isn't strictly true. A more accurate description would be you are what you absorb. By now, we should all know the benefits of eating more vegetables – but let's be realistic, not many of us can eat two heads of broccoli, a bag of carrots, and five lettuces every day. Even if eating large amounts of vegetables were sustainable day in and day out, your poor digestive system would be working overtime to break it all down. Fortunately, juicing allows us to bypass this whole process and those nutrients are easier to absorb when juiced than they are if you try to eat your way through the same amount in solid form.

In solid food, fiber is important to aid digestion, but because juicing is a liquid, it's okay that most of the fiber is removed by the juicing machine. Keep in mind that this is a balance. I appreciate that if the juice doesn't taste good, some people will be reluctant to drink it. But we don't want to fall into the trap of adding too much fruit, either. Once the fiber is removed from fruit you should really think of it as liquid sugar. This is really important to remember. Moderation is always key, more so if you are dealing with a particular low grade fungal or bacterial infection.

There are lots of juicers on the market, some big, some small, some are affordable and some can be darn right expensive. Some are quality built and some are junk. Some juicers will outperform others and the tradeoff for doing so can be more time spent cleaning up. So before you rush out and buy one, know that the best juicer to buy is the one you will use. Even a top of the line juicer is useless if it sits in the cupboard because it takes too long to clean.

In my humble opinion, owning a juicer is better than having money in the bank. For sure, buying a juicer can be an investment, but there are few things in this life worth investing in more than your health – and let's be clear, illness ain't cheap!

Finding the right juicer for your needs is important. I urge you to check out a guy by the name of John who runs the YouTube channel DiscountJuicers.com. John has an unbiased passion for putting juicers through their paces. If anyone can tell you which juicer will fill your needs, it's John. Personally, I like the Omega VSJ843. As a first juicer, it's got a decent warranty and it's pretty simple to use. Ideally I would have liked the excess pulp to be a little dryer, but hey, the tradeoff is that compared to some other juicers it's relatively easy to clean.

By adding selective fruits (in moderation) juicing can be a pleasurable experience. No seriously, get this right and you can even get the kids to drink their greens! Think apples, with a hint of ginger, mixed with blueberries, celery, and lime, perhaps add a hint of fresh mint, parsley, or even kale. Huh? Just relax, kale is nothing more than angry lettuce, when the amount of kale in the juice is right you won't even taste it.

Before you diss the kale, know that it's loaded with thiamin, riboflavin, folate, iron, magnesium, and phosphorus. It's also a good source of vitamins A, C, K, B6, as well as calcium, potassium, copper, and manganese. Compared to popping a pill can you see why the health benefits surrounding juicing are unique? Juicing drives nutrients into the digestive system while at the same time packing a nutritional EZ punch.

Some people run juicing alongside their current diet, and some use it as a standalone way of intermittent fasting, the benefits of which were covered in Chapter 15 (Hit the Reset Button). The trick to juicing is to make your green juice taste good and the good news is there are now hundreds of free juicing blogs to help give you additional support.

It's kinda difficult to narrow it down because there are soooo many good ones out there. I guess Kimberly Snyder would be one of the better known ones. Kimberly not only radiates with health; she also has a genuine passion for helping people. Her website has all kinds of wonderful information. There is a link to her in another chapter, or if you are rolling as a paperback homie, check out KimberlySnyder.com

Over the years I've always tried to get my information from a diverse pool of people. I find this helps give my research a healthy balance. So when it comes to juicing blogs, I'd also like to give a big shout out to Dan McDonald.

Of all the admirable qualities a man can possess, overcoming adversity is the one I admire most. Lord knows, Dan's life hasn't always been easy and on the surface he might seem like an unlikely health guru. A former drug addict whose mom died when he was just three years old, Dan was then raised by an extremely abusive father.

With over 1500 unscripted YouTube videos under his belt, Dan turned that adversity into something uniquely positive. For me, Dan's honesty is deeply refreshing. There is no slick editing and in some of Dan's early videos he makes mistakes, sometimes says weird shit, and simply carries on. What you see is what you get, which is often a man wearing no shirt but looking great! His show, The Life Regenerator, can be found on YouTube. Check it out.

WHEATGRASS

When talking about juicing I'd be doing you a great disservice if I didn't tip my hat to the subject of wheatgrass. Wheatgrass juice packs a real nutritional punch, and it's something I used to grow. The vitamins and minerals found in just two ounces of freshly squeezed juice equal three pounds of organic vegetables!

Wheatgrass juice is approximately 70% crude chlorophyll which is nearly identical to the hemoglobin found in red blood cells.

Chlorophyll in wheatgrass juice has been shown to increase the function of the heart, help the vascular system, the intestines, and the lungs. It's also said to speed up blood circulation, cleanse the blood of waste, lower high blood pressure, and stimulate healthy tissue cell. Wheatgrass is rich in vitamin K, which is essential in bone formation.

Wheatgrass juice also contains 90 out of 102 vitamins, minerals, and nutrients, including vitamins A, B (niacin, riboflavin, thiamine), C, E, and K, as well as choline, calcium, chlorine, iron, magnesium, phosphorus, potassium, sodium, sulfur, cobalt, and zinc, not to mention twenty amino acids and about thirty enzymes. I know, right? It beats taking that harsh multi-vitamin.

If you can keep a houseplant alive then growing wheatgrass is totally doable. The grass grows quickly and in seven to ten days will be approximately 8" tall. Then you cut the grass and turn it into juice via a hand cranked juicer.

Although wheatgrass takes a little more effort, it is another good tool to have under your belt.

Wheatgrass juice can also be bought in some juice bars but it should ALWAYS be consumed fresh. There are lots of books out there on wheatgrass and the one I like best is The Wheatgrass Book by Ann Wigmore. It's a small, well-written and easy to understand book.

MAX GERSON

Finally, for anyone looking to overcome serious illness the Gerson Therapy is a natural treatment that activates the body's extraordinary ability to heal itself through an organic, plant-based diet, raw juices, coffee enemas (yup you heard me right), and natural supplements.

With its whole-body approach to healing, the Gerson Therapy is a powerful treatment to have in the toolbox. If you find yourself in a tight medical spot there is also a movie on YouTube called The Beautiful Truth that covers the Gerson Therapy in more detail.
Dr. Max Gerson first developed this therapy in the 1930s, initially as a treatment for his own debilitating migraines and eventually as a treatment for a wide range of degenerative diseases. Over the years many people have claimed to have used this therapy in the fight against cancer. Dr. Gerson's work was later carried on by his now 95-year-old daughter Charlotte.

What did we learn from this chapter?

Keeping an open mind allows you to explore practices that may have a significant impact on your life, for example seeing liquids in a different way. Juicing is truly transformative. Health is an investment, not an expense.

Homework:
- If you haven't read my first book, please feel free to check it out on Amazon. https://www.amazon.com/dp/B071JRBRW6

PART 1

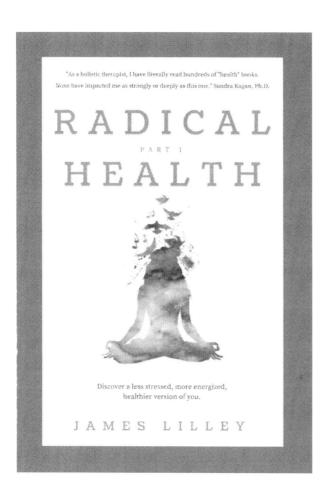

Chapter 13

YOU HAVE A GIFT

Growing up in government housing as I did wasn't always perfect but it was always interesting. At times people were perhaps a little too quick to settle their differences the old fashioned way, standing toe to toe with clenched fists, thus ensuring the ointment of life always had an element of grit to it. In the middle of this madness I was extremely fortunate to have someone in my life who was respected by all.

Dad was one of those unusual people who could turn his hand to anything and do it well. He could fix the toaster and the car; he was a meticulous maker of intricate things, he even knew his way around a boxing ring, and he could play the guitar. With his magical tricks and witty jokes, he could entertain a room full of people with ease.

At the age of fifty he started running in marathons and, just for good measure, he always crossed the finish line by doing a forward roll – in spite of his bad back. They say you can't teach an old dog new tricks but he once rewired a whole house to an impeccably high standard and then grew a prize vegetable garden from seed!

Over the years he developed an uncanny knack for being right and people often came to ask his advice. He lived his life free of debt and spent money wisely. He never drank and he never swore.

And yes, he could even fix the TV set and the radio, but Dad's greatest gift was his handwritten notes which always carried a beautiful majestic flow.

Writing seemed to light a fire deep inside him and in his spare time he would leave informative notes for anybody who would read them.

172

Before leaving for work he often left Mom a page-long letter, and when eBay first came along he spent an hour writing the most eloquent description just to sell an old coat. It's fair to say Dad's writing was not only his gift, it was his passion. The problem was he didn't know it, and so he settled for less.

So for thirty-five years he fed his family by driving a double-decker bus which due to his precise nature, always ran on time. His bus driver uniform was always neatly pressed in a certain way, and his clean, polished shoes stood out from a meter away.

Dad never skipped a day of work, not even when he was ill. With an unblemished driving record that stretched more than three decades, his number one goal was to deliver people safely to their destination. It's fair to say he was honest and friendly with everyone he met.

Late one night a man boarded and left his wallet behind. The wallet quickly found its way back to its owner. Another night a drunk spat in his face – he wasn't quite as easy to trace. If you asked my dad why he drove a big red bus he would joke, "It's an easy job, my load walks on and walks off." He tried to find a positive in every situation.

Dad was gifted in so many ways and I'll never know why such a meticulous mind spent eight hours a day driving a big red bus. He sometimes wrote such eloquent handwritten letters that I'd catch myself rushing through them. If only I'd known back then I would have said, "Hey Dad, why don't you write down all those practical tips that you know?" He often told us things like, "Never buy a house at the bottom of the hill."

Earlier this week the local news ran a story about a street that had been flooded out, except of course for the house that stood at the top of the hill. Sadly, Dad's not here anymore so my question to you is this.

What's your passion and why aren't you doing it? In this chapter we hope to find out.

To better understand ourselves it's important to understand our psychological traits. Are you introverted or extroverted? Do you lead with your head or your heart? Are you goal oriented or people orientated?

The Swiss psychiatrist and psychoanalyst Carl Jung founded analytical psychology. He believed our distinguishing characteristics have a tendency to fit into four basic personality types. For ease of understanding, Jung color-coded these four categories using the colors yellow, red, blue, and green. See if you can recognize yourself in any of them. Ready?

YELLOW

Yellows like to be around people and are very much the life and soul of the party. They are sociable, expressive, imaginative, and enthusiastic. They are also informal, optimistic, and animated. Yellows have creative imaginations that can sometimes run away with them as they are very fast paced thinkers. Yellows don't like to be slowed down with intricate details or formalities.

RED

Reds like to take control. They are strong-willed, fast-paced thinkers, risk takers, purposeful, less patient, overtly competitive, formal, and rational. They don't like small talk and prefer people get straight to the point, which is why this description is short.

BLUE

Cool blues are deep thinkers, analytical in nature, very detail focused and formal in their thinking. They are deliberate, systematic, precise, and pay great attention to detail. They like things in their place and have excellent time management skills. They are much slower paced than the reds or yellows. Blues like to have all the facts and then logically put together a suitable answer. Blues don't like to be rushed into things or be disorganized.

GREEN

Greens are laid back, relaxed, and patient. They are easy to get along with and informal in their approach. They are social and focus more on relationships and may at times come across as emotional. They are much slower paced in their thinking and are very democratic people. They are very understanding and agreeable. Greens sometimes make the perfect go between for Reds and Yellows, who are much faster paced. They also act as the facilitator to conflicts. Greens don't like to be pushed or put on the spot.

Did you see yourself in any of these four groups? How about family members or your partner?

When we choose a partner we are sometimes drawn to personality types that are opposite us. We can then spend our whole lives being driven crazy by them, and they us!

Knowing what color best suits your partner can help unlock those complicated interpersonal relations. If you want to show your affection to a green, give them a hug, if you want to show affection to a red, offer to complete a task in record time. Knowing what makes a person tick is halfway to a lasting relationship.

Understanding ourselves helps us better understand our role in the workplace. When we are happy in our work we are less stressed. All too often we base our entire working lives on our academic achievements rather than taking into account our specific personality traits.

Knowing who and what you are may help you fit into a job you enjoy, although it seems quite odd that we are told to choose a career before we can even legally buy a beer. If you are currently stuck in a job that you dislike this chapter may prove particularly insightful. The good news is it's never too late to change.

> The privilege of a lifetime is being who you are.
> – Joseph Campbell

When you look at the diagram below there are no right or wrong answers, only relevant ones. It's not uncommon to find yourself 80% dominant in one color and 20% in another. Check which category best suits your personality best and then see how it could be put to good use in a working environment.

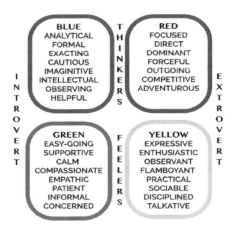

Once you have a basic understanding of these four categories life becomes less enigmatic and even teenage kids become easier to understand. Keep in mind if you are hoping to ground a blue teenager be sure to give them all the reasons, if you are going to ground a red teenager give them the fastest way to become ungrounded. Understand that a green teenager needs compassion and good luck clipping the wings of a social yellow!

If we relate these colors back to the work place, can you see a blue introvert working in customer sales? Nah, I don't think so. How about a yellow extrovert working in sales? Hmm, maybe. How about a fiery red dentist? Nah, I think I'll take my chances with the more supportive green one.

My point is this: the only way to do great work is to love what you do. If you hate your job, it shows. Maybe the real reason you dislike your job is because you are not being true to yourself.

FIND YOUR GIFT

No matter which color you identify with, you, my friend, have a gift somewhere deep inside you. Everyone does. Your job is to find it. A clue might be that subject that you love to talk about. Once you know where to look, your gift is actually pretty easy to find. What's the one thing that you do that seems easy or obvious to you, while others may struggle or muddle their way through? Congrats, that would be your gift.

> The meaning of life is to find your gift;
> the purpose of life is to give it away.
> – Picasso

Once you have your gift, own it, nurture it, fight for it. It's the fastest way to a meaningful life. All too often we are told we must run with the pack, swim with the current, or follow the crowd.

Often we are conditioned to think it's too late to change; you can't do this, obey the rules, accept the limitations imposed by others. Life is good at getting us to conform the same way my dad did for most of his working life.

Do what you love and all good things will come. This should be easy to do right? Meh, not so fast. Let's not forget some of us were educated in decaying inner city schools and taught from an early age to think inside the box – such impressionable young minds all programmed to expect and accept less.

> People will forget what you said, people will forget what you did, but people will never forget how you made them feel.
> – Maya Angelou

Unfortunately, that last quote strikes a chord with my school experience. Standing in the corner facing the wall can be a deeply humiliating experience. Once used to shame those who failed to grasp basic information, it also served to suppress the human spirit. I don't ever recall my teachers every saying, "Follow your dream, do what you love, we believe in you!" Instead we were forced to learn about algebra.

BROKEN TOILETS AND BAD KNEES

As a result, I am sometimes caught up in self-doubt and conflict. Like my dad before me, I've spent much of my life doing work that perhaps I wasn't destined to do. Over the past few years I've been used to earning my money the hard way – with my hands. Give me two young guys with strong backs and I can fix your house from the ground up – although these days I find it less stressful to work quietly on my own.

Yeah, that's right, I'm the guy without an education whom you call to come clean up your yard or fix that broken gutter.

You see, I'm still fighting for my gift – even this minute as I write this, I'm still tormented with an internal debate about whether I should abandon this foolish idea of writing this book and just stick to being a construction worker. In the winter months when work is thin on the ground, I either read more or I write. But it might surprise you to know that over the course of the previous two chapters I've also been busy painting the side of someone's house, repairing a toilet, and hanging a new door for a customer.

Between construction gigs, I can be found with a small notebook in my pocket containing a collection of thoughts that I reshape daily until they become something interesting or new. Like my dad, I refused to believe old dogs are incapable of learning new things.

> The capacity to learn is a gift;
> The ability to learn is a skill;
> The willingness to learn is a choice.
> – Brian Herbert

While carrying out those recent home repairs, I noticed the elderly homeowner had a problem with his knee. To fix his toilet, I replaced the inlet valve, to fix his knee I suggested he apply dimethyl-sulfoxide (DMSO) directly to the area twice a day and then refrain from eating all reactive foods in the nightshade family for one month.

From the look on his face I guess he thought handymen only fixed toilets. Fortunately, he was in enough obvious pain to see past my overalls and within a week the treatment had taken most of the inflammation out of the joint. Either way, my customer was grateful even if he was a little mystified as to why he could suddenly walk unaided again.

As a rule, I generally keep my thoughts to myself for fear of being misunderstood. I was once updating a kitchen for a customer whom I overheard complaining of eye pain. When I suggested she immediately get herself checked out by a doctor, she scoffed at my advice. I know, right? What could the handyman possibly know about optic neuritis?

Maybe I just see things differently; I guess I've always been a bit of a square peg in a round hole. Whenever I'm asked the dreaded question what I do for work, I cannot claim to be a writer without a published word to my name, although this is how I spend my evenings. I cannot claim to be a nutritionist, although I do have an understanding of nutrition. I cannot claim to be formally educated, and yet I am not uneducated. So I usually reply, "I'm just a handyman." This is generally met with a silent nod as if they already know my type. It seems that people like to pigeonhole us as a way of helping them work out who we are. I'm currently toying with the idea of telling people I blow up bridges just to gauge their reaction.

So by now you are probably now wondering how does a fifty-two year old, often underemployed handyman with no previous medical experience come to know all this stuff? It's called unbending persistence, although if you were paying close attention you already know this from Chapter 2.

It's true that where there is a will there is always a way. When something is important to us we either find a way or we find an excuse, and nobody cares how good the excuses are for not doing something! To some, I'm sure I must appear quite odd as much of this book has been written while living out of a suitcase and there are times when the only quiet place I have to type up my notes is parked in my vehicle.

With hindsight maybe this year wasn't the best time to try and write this book. In recent weeks attempting to balance work, family life, and find a new home has become a challenge. When I pick up my tool belt I can expect to get paid on Fridays, when I pick up my pen it becomes a source of friction.

I'm as human as the next guy and when something becomes stressful I also hear that uneasy loop playing over in my mind – Give up, go back to what you know, you shouldn't be doing this. Or my personal favorite –This is a waste of good time.

In my darkest hour when I was on the verge of saying, to hell with it all, I quit, hope came from another unpublished writer, my daughter. Her simple note below has been driving me to see this project through to the end.

Dad,
I want to remind you of something. You're not writing this book for you, you are writing this book for people who have little hope left, for people as ill as you were, who have no way to get out. You're writing this book for your kids and your kids' kids. You're writing this book because you said you wanted to help people. You wanted to write this book so that nobody had to go through what you went through.

You are writing this book for a reason, for a purpose. You were meant to be a writer, not a carpenter, not a mechanic, not a handyman, you were meant to mean something, to change something, to be an inspiration to people who have none left. There's a fire in you to write, a certain creativity. You were meant to be a writer and I just wanted to tell you that. P.S. I Love you. X

It seems that regardless of my situation, this book isn't going to leave me alone until it's written so I have no business quitting.

What did we learn from this chapter?

Often we are conditioned to believe our foolish dreams are too big and we should give up on them. But the simple truth is you need only to find your gift and then use it to do what you were put here to do.

People generally fit into four basic groups, knowing which one you belong to will help in both your career and your relationships. This in turn helps reduce stress which makes you more acidic, a subject we keep coming back to. To have any chance of inner peace we should first know who and what we are.

Homework: you can see Dr. Jacobs talk about the healing power of DMSO (Dimethyl sulfoxide) for yourself by watching the short video clip below. Keep in mind there is no big money to be made from DMSO which is perhaps why some people like to jump all over it.

DMSO is sometimes used to help protect delicate donor organs while they are in on their way to transplant patients. The FDA also approved DMSO for the treatment of interstitial cystitis suggesting it has a valid place in medicine. Am I saying DMOS is right for everyone? Nope, never did say that, but for someone facing the surgeon's scalpel and a 50k bill for a knee operation, it sometimes pays to have a few options on the table (or to keep you off the table).

The video clip below is taken from 60 minutes and although it's a little dated, the information remains as valid as ever.
https://www.youtube.com/watch?v=H_szhaOS9V4

Chapter 14

WOBBLY FOOD

While I haven't always been a country boy, it's fair to say I've always been a home boy. Over several months we spent so much time wandering across Europe looking for a new home that the adventure aspect of living out of a suitcase wore thin. All the upheaval brought a new heaviness to my soul and I began to miss my orderly life, my OCD vegetable garden, and a familiar place to hang my hat.

Living in a state of limbo became too stressful and, unable to find a new place to call home, we found ourselves back in the city in a rented apartment. It's fair to say this has been something of an adjustment, but compared to another day of uncertainty I am, for the moment, gladly embracing my new concrete garden.

Being out of my comfort zone will no doubt come through in these final few chapters. Perhaps it's refreshing to learn that there are days when we all struggle and this path to clean living isn't always going to be easy. Even the best laid plans can misfire on us. As John Lennon once said, "Life is what happens while you are busy making other plans," although you never know because he also said, "I am the egg-man, I am the walrus."

Keep in mind that for much of the past decade I've been living in a small rural community, growing my own food, and heating my house with wood cut from my own land. Now I find myself living in an apartment where heat is available at the touch of a button which has the magnetic allure of a new tire in a monkey park. I've been used to preparing for cooler nights six months in advance. That usually involved dropping a tree early in the spring (to give it time to dry out) before splitting it with an axe in the fall.

Chopping down a tree may sound like work, but in many respects my life was much easier when I didn't have to worry about paying for heat. I also had access to a local freshwater stream, an organic garden, and I had gotten to know all the local farmers by name.

Although I grew up in the city, coming back has me feeling a bit like a fish out of water. The tranquility of listening to a babbling brook has suddenly been replaced with whoever lives upstairs walking across my ceiling.

As I struggle to adjust back into city life, while at the same time living under somebody else's rules, I've also taken to sucking water out of plastic bottles and my once pristine diet has fallen. It's not that I'm being lazy. Shipping everything across the Atlantic after we'd sold our tiny homestead made no economic sense. But suddenly being disconnected from the things I had come to rely on has shown me that it is not always easy to maintain a healthy lifestyle on the fly.

Over the years I've spent enough time listening to online health gurus to form the opinion that most are genuinely nice people who never misplace a nutritional foot as they are carried from podcast to podcast on the shoulders of infidels. Alas, I can no longer pledge my allegiance to such high standards so I'm afraid you are going to have to tolerate a little more of my disappointing honesty. I'm a real person and sometimes I mess up.

Last night I found myself ill prepared, hungry, and staring into an open food cupboard where the only thing looking back at me was a lone box of cereal. I'm not going to pretend I'm perfect or even explain why it was there, but in a moment of weakness I ate the whole stupid box. I know, right? What's next, Flakka?

At the moment I seem to be backsliding faster than a speeding ticket. This morning I even caught a family member trying to eat yellow Jell-

O for breakfast. The fact that yellow Jell-O has to be made ahead of time is what worries me the most. It was a premeditated attempt to eat a food group that wobbles and now suddenly I'm the bad guy.

It would seem that at any given point in this life, we are all either swimming with the current, floating on a log, or drowning. Today it feels as if I'm spluttering on a little more water than usual.

As unwelcome as this experience is, it's also inspired me to write these remaining chapters with fresh eyes. So, while I'm over here taking a hit for the team, here are a couple more home truths. You probably won't like hearing them, but I'm going to spill the beans anyways. I've recently rediscovered that unless you have access to your own year-round organic garden or limitless funds for your own private chef, there is going to come a point when you find yourself standing in a sterile supermarket feeling overwhelmed by it all, am I right?

For those of us struggling to find organic food grown by one armed monks or who have fallen off the no-gluten wagon, know that we are not the first nor will we be the last. There is no point in beating ourselves up over it; tomorrow is another day and we will pick ourselves up, dust ourselves off, and go again. If this is you, take a deep breath and know that it's going to be okay, okay? Let's draw a line under today and begin moving forward.

Whenever I fall from nutritional grace, I find it helpful to ask: why the hell am I doing this, anyway? Maybe, like me, you are just sick of being sick. Maybe you are simply tired of being tired. The only right answer is an answer that motivates you. Perhaps you simply want that elusive summer beach body to show off, or you need more energy to play Frisbee with the grandkids.

This whole finding what motivates you thing is pretty important – fear, pain, bikinis, accountability, family, and even recognition are all powerful motivators. Knowing which one motivates you can make the difference between success and failure.

Find the driving force behind why you do what you do – that has to be your reason for wanting more health and less sickness. You don't have to make this complicated; the right answer is always going to be the one that motivates you. One way to turn that thought into a powerful commitment is to write it down.

NOTE THE EXCUSES

Whatever it is that's motivating you, know that better health starts with what goes on the end of your fork. You might think that's waaaay too simple, but it's actually true. It's important to be honest with yourself here. Are there any patterns that may be creeping in – like you didn't have time to cook, or you couldn't find the right ingredients?

Then ask yourself whether these genuine reasons or whether you let a handful of excuses trip you up? You know the ones I'm talking about, those lame excuses like the kids made me do it, everyone else was doing it, or my personal favorite, "I thought I could have just one." Yeah right, damn you hard licorice Scotty dogs.

We would do well to remember there is no shame in falling down. The shame is to keep falling down in the exact same place! Knowing our excuses in advance helps us see the same repetitive pattern. You really want to own this one and sometimes writing down three reasons why we fell off the nutritional wagon forces us to acknowledge these are areas that trip us up.

So far we have our motivating reason for doing this and our excuses for not doing it, if you have your paper and pencil handy what say we go the extra mile?

Ready?

Even though we may have fallen off the wagon, starting today let's set five ground rules that we absolutely refuse to budge on even on days when all else fails. Setting a new baseline makes it harder to fall below the standard you deserve. For me, I'm going to say no matter how dysfunctional my current environment gets, I won't drink soda, I won't eat white bread, I won't drink milk, I won't eat any more licorice candy, and I absolutely, point blank, refuse to eat yellow Jell-O for breakfast! I know, right? Let's hope somebody just browsing the book section didn't turn to this paragraph first.

Once we have our shit together let's get back on the horse. To help us stay in the saddle I have some breakfast tips coming in the next chapter. They probably won't win any culinary awards, but they may help you survive meal times when all the low hanging organic fruit has been replaced with concrete. The good news is the morning after the night before breakfast is super easy to get right.

What did we learn from this chapter?

We all mess up – own it. Quit whining about it and try again. If you still need pizza check below.

Homework: to help you stay on track, check out this short video by Kimberly Snyder. Here Kimberly offers simple step by step advice for those looking to find a healthy pizza! If you get the opportunity, please feel free to mention where you found her information.

https://www.facebook.com/KimberlySnyderCN/videos/15109618855
93465/

Chapter 15

WHAT THE HELL DO I EAT FOR BREAKFAST?

It's often said that breakfast is the most important meal of the day, this is the one piece of mainstream advice I think we can all agree on, alas not for the reasons you may be thinking. Breakfast is the most important meal because getting this wrong can set up failure for the rest of the day.

Starting the day off with a boxed cereal containing dried fruit, grains, added sugar, topped with a splash of cow's milk is sure to promote inflammation and a sugar spike even before the day has begun. Sheesh, talk about a cereal killer.

Even worse, many think swiping a banana off the counter as we head through the door is a "healthy" breakfast option. But ask yourself, when you eat this way, how's your hunger and energy level at about 11:30 a.m?

You may have noticed that sugar has become rampant in this world, and so too has illness. We can now walk around any supermarket and find fruit (another form of sugar) even when it's out of season. Let's keep in mind that not only does fruit turn to sugar, so too does protein, as do carbohydrates, as does fruit juice, so the last thing we need are more manmade sugars like sodas, cookies, and a million other additives adding to the sugar burden. As Nobel Prize winner Otto Warburg pointed out waaaaay back in 1931, cancer cells need sugar to replicate.

Now we know what breakfast isn't, let's be clear about what breakfast is. Break-fast literally means, "breaking the fast" and it's usually the first meal we eat after sleeping. For some of us, it could have been twelve plus hours since our last meal, although this isn't necessarily a bad thing. Here's why.

Given the average breakfast choices of cereal, toast, or fruit we might be better off eating no breakfast at all. This alone is an interesting concept. The body is smart. Ever notice how the first thing to leave us when we feel ill is our appetite? The body automatically sends us into intermittent fasting mode. This is a process that actually dates back to biblical times and even the modern day science behind fasting is pretty mind blowing.

Once again, I could easily fill up the rest of this chapter with scientific references to support this notion, but life is short and there is absolutely no time left to waste. Let's summarize by saying that intermittent fasting can (and does) help with everything from cellular repair to human growth hormone, from gene repair to improved insulin levels, yada, yada, yada. But for my money, the most interesting aspect of intermittent fasting is that it increases energy.

While I'm not advocating any one diet over another, many aspects of the ketogenic diet seem to fit this concept quite well because it flips the body into fat burning mode rather than using glucose as the primary fuel. And please note that I'm not saying other diets can't work. There are some people who obviously thrive on a vegetarian diet while others do not. The idea is to try to keep an open mind, and if your health is in a ditch don't be afraid to try new things. The only diet I can't imagine people thriving on is the Standard American Diet which, despite its name, has now been exported to many other countries around the globe. So SAD.

When we push back on the morning urge to eat sugary carbs two things happen: first, we aren't being slowed down by excess sugars and second, the body is encouraged to burn fat in the form of ketones. Ketones, as you may recall from an earlier chapter, are produced in the liver during periods of low food intake. The body then uses them as an alternative fuel source. The benefits of burning ketones for energy are many, and absent a recognized eating disorder, pushing back on carbs isn't too big an issue for most of us.

Either way, in this chapter you will find seven breakfast ideas to help you break away from all those sugary carbs. These ideas are so simple even I can do them and best of all there are no calories to count. The trick is to play around with these ideas until you find one that works best for you. Ideally, in the morning we could slip into intermittent fasting mode but if that's a little too rock and roll for you, then let's kick around with the idea of increasing our intake of healthy fat while reducing our overall carb intake.

BREAKFAST IDEA #1, THE BULLET

Up until now I've been pretty good at taking things away from you and your reward for sticking with me is about to be paid. How would you like a breakfast that gently lifts brain fog and gives you more energy? Better still, it can make you feel good and, in the process, you won't even feel hungry until midafternoon. Welcome to the world of butter-coffee or "Bulletproof" coffee!

Bulletproof coffee is the brain child of Dave Asprey. Dave is one of those curious people who refuse to accept illness as an acceptable destination and while he makes no claim to have invented intermittent fasting, he certainly came up with a novel idea for a better way to do it.

First, let's address why some data suggests that drinking coffee is bad for you. It might help to know that whenever you read a study relating to coffee, the quality of that coffee is rarely taken into account. This is huge because the difference between regular coffee and high quality coffee is the same as the difference between night and day. When the two are treated as the same, results are always going to be skewed. Make no mistake, Bulletproof coffee is an upgraded version of the stuff sold in the average coffee shop.

Ever wonder why your cup of Joe makes you feel good and then a few hours later you crash? It's all to do with where and when the beans were harvested. Mycotoxins are a form of mold that the naked eye cannot see, once they get into the coffee harvesting process they are thought to be the reason for that crash.

So yes, finding the right bean is key, and beans grown at higher elevations in Central America are less likely to be affected by such molds. For that reason, stay well away from blends that are almost certainly going to include beans from lower down on the mountain. There are lots of options out there and Dave Asprey himself sells a brand of coffee that has been carefully screened for such molds.

Coffee sometimes gets a bad rap for stressing the adrenal glands. This is something I am well aware of, but again it's more likely to be lower grade coffee so let's not be in a rush to throw the baby out with the bathwater. If you are suffering from any type of adrenal dysfunction, supplementing with cordyceps has a wide range of health benefits. Cordyceps have adaptogenic properties which is something we will look into later.

Research shows its powerful effect to improve kidney, adrenal, brain, pancreatic and hormonal health. You may also find relief from a wonderfully helpful herb by the name of ashwagandha, both of these supplements have adaptogenic qualities, an important subject I'd like to try to squeeze in before this book ends.

Use Bulletproof coffee as an alternative to eating energy-zapping cereals for breakfast. I've been doing this myself for the past few months and trust me, Bulletproof butter-coffee hits the spot, it's something to try at least once and see how you do.

The science behind Bulletproof coffee is impressive, but more important, this is a tip that works. Bulletproof coffee is easy to make, but in order to pull it off you need three key ingredients.

1. A high quality coffee bean.

2. MCT oil which is short for Medium-Chain Triglycerides. MCT oil is a form of saturated fatty acid that has numerous health benefits ranging from improved cognitive function to better weight management.

3. Grass fed butter such as Kerrigold.

Please note: Inferior substitutions simply will not work.

Bulletproof coffee has plenty of good fats that come in the form of MCT oil and butter from grass-fed cows. If you feel good doing it, then keep going, if you feel worse, don't hesitate to stop and try something else. I hope by now the take-home message is loud and clear: there is no one size fits all. Don't be shy in trying out other options until you find something here that works for you.

A deeper reference to these key ingredients can be found in this helpful how-to video by Dave Asprey himself. To learn how to make Bulletproof coffee, click the link below.

https://www.youtube.com/watch?v=4YjLMdx3YZY

Dave can also be found on his podcast "Bulletproof radio" which is something I regularly tune into.

BREAKFAST IDEA #2, BACON SALAD

If bulletproof coffee didn't do it for you, then this next breakfast suggestion is relatively quick and easy to make, the idea here is to give you a few workable tools as opposed to being a culinary tour de force.

So our mornings look to be leaning toward the higher fat and lower carb spectrum. This leads us neatly into bacon salad.

To save time, simply pick up a box of mixed salad from the store. These types of pre-made salads aren't perfect, but they do cut down on time and waste. Bonus points if it's organic. If not, don't panic, just do the best you can. Know that this breakfast is a step up from that boxed cereal and it really doesn't take much to prepare, it's also going to help save us from a sugar crash later in the day.

I'm not going to micro-manage you on the bacon, you know how you like your bacon cooked better than I do, so long as you aren't cooking with bad fats. While the bacon is cooking grab a clean plate and throw a handful of mixed salad onto it. Add a squirt of apple cider vinegar and a pinch of salt. As soon as the bacon is done, add it to the salad and eat. The simplicity of this meal means food triggers are kept to a minimum.

If you have it, you can also pour a little MCT oil over the salad, again this ensures your breakfast starts with plenty of good fats which will keep you from feeling deprived throughout the day.

As with anything new, be aware of how this makes you feel. While most people will experience a positive health benefit from adding MCT oil, I can think of at least one person I know who seems to do better without it. If your regular breakfast is usually cereal, then you may need to give your body a chance to adjust to this cleaner, leaner way of eating breakfast. Sometimes it just takes a little time.

You may be wondering why eggs are missing from the bacon salad. While it may be true that eggs are nutritious, there are many, many people who react badly to them. For now, let's try this breakfast without the eggs and then perhaps a month down the road add them in and closely monitor how you feel. As mentioned in a previous chapter, not everyone will roll on the floor and turn blue; some reactions will be delayed and subtle, such as general fatigue.

BREAKFAST IDEA #3, GO-AVOCADO

Technically a fruit, avocados have a lot of vegetable-type qualities. Avocados are nutritionally dense and a better source of potassium than bananas. Do I like avocado? No, I can't stand the damned things but it's another form of good fat and if it keeps me on my feet I'll eat them.

Although the idea is to limit fruit for breakfast, adding a little lime juice and a few blueberries makes an avocado more palatable. You can even add a pinch of Himalayan sea salt for added kick. Avocados come loaded with heart-healthy monounsaturated fatty acids. Need more fiber? Go avocado.

BREAKFAST IDEA #4, BUDWIG

If we haven't found your thang yet, then rest assured, the Budwig breakfast is an interesting one. This idea is accredited to German biochemist Johanna Budwig who was also a highly respected pharmacist and held degrees in physics and chemistry. She lived to be ninety-five and was nominated seven times for the Nobel Peace Prize. Why am I bothering to mention all this? Obviously Johanna Budwig was a very smart lady and her simple Budwig diet has been suggested by some to be a powerful protocol for certain cancers. You can find more information relating to this on a website called Cancer Tutor. Am I saying this is a cure for cancer? Nope, never did that, never would, just thought you might find the information behind the Budwig diet interesting reading.

The reason I've included the Budwig breakfast here is because it's simple to make and it tastes good. For this little party piece, you are going to need some organic flaxseed oil and some organic cottage cheese (even better would be goat's milk quark or sheep's milk quark if you can find it). You can also add some berries to make it taste good, preferably berries that are in season.

Here's how you make it:

Place 6 tablespoons of organic cottage cheese in a mixing bowl.

Add 3 tablespoons good quality flaxseed oil.

(Only buy QUALITY flaxseed oil from a store that keeps it fresh in a refrigerator and always check the sell-by date.)

Add 2 tablespoons freshly ground flaxseeds

Whisk it all together with a simple immersion hand blender and you are good to go.

Optional: if you want to make it more palatable, throw in a handful of berries or ground nuts.

This breakfast is simple, filling, and unless you are dairy sensitive, it's super healthy!

BREAKFAST IDEA #5, OKAY-OATS

There are times when you may feel a need to refuel with a few carbs. Gluten-free oats are a much better option than toast. It's important to steer away from mass produced oats as they are almost certainly cross-contaminated with gluten during processing. Plain oats can be made more interesting by adding nuts, berries, or a shake of cinnamon. Buying plain oats from a health food store ensures you aren't subjecting your digestive system to added sugars.

Resist buying instant oats which usually come loaded with sugar. Instead, soak plain oats in a bowl of water overnight. In the morning simply strain them and heat them in a saucepan with a little fresh water or almond milk. Viola! They are as fast as instant oats without all the additives. Oats are also quick to make and a good source of fiber.

BREAKFAST IDEA # 6, MINI-MASTER

Some mornings you might not feel up to eating a big breakfast, especially when it's warm out, if this is you, simply make a mini master cleanse drink. This drink will not only help to detoxify your liver it can also keep hunger at bay for a few hours. Generally speaking, this works best with room temperature water.

Add 3 tablespoons of fresh lemon juice to twelve ounces of water. Mix in a teaspoon (or less) of pure, dark maple syrup and a pinch of cayenne pepper. Shake and drink.

A month from now your liver will thank you. Don't be afraid to mix this up a little. In recent months I've been doing this without the maple syrup and I'm still here to tell the tale.

This last one is a great go to breakfast for those cold winter mornings. It's also quick to make and ideal for those in need of a little more mental energy. Best of all, you only need seven ingredients which you may or may not already have. If you don't, they can be found in your local health food store and they seem to last forever. To save time I'm just going to jump in and tell you how to make this, but if you want to know why this works, or what brands I use, be sure to check out my Facebook page (details are at the end of this book). This one is my own recipe and it pays to remember there are 7 ingredients, enjoy!

Okay, grab one medium saucepan and throw in one tablespoon of raw cocoa powder. Next add one teaspoon of powdered Turmeric. Now add a quarter spoon of Himalayan sea salt. Freshly grind one stick of cinnamon and throw that in too. Next add a pinch of organic cayenne powder. Add 16oz of water and bring to boil. Once boiled allow to simmer for 5 mins. While simmering add two tablespoons of Kerrigold butter and wait for it to melt. Now whisk it all together with a hand blender. Last but not least, add one tablespoon of MCT oil to a large mug (not the saucepan). Now, pour the liquid from the saucepan into the mug, give it a stir and hey presto, your Healthy-Alfie is ready to drink! You can also add a little unsweetened almond milk if you feel so inclined.

What did we learn from this chapter?

We are all different, what works for one person might not work for another and it's important to be open to new ideas. The breakfast options in this section are pretty basic but they will outperform cereal or toast.

Homework: for some unique nutritional insight, check out Dr. Berg on YouTube. Dr. Berg makes interesting short videos and I always come away learning something new.

Link: https://www.youtube.com/watch?v=5vIoHR7J24I

Chapter 16

WHAT THE HELL DO I EAT FOR LUNCH?

The key to making any of this work is to try to plan ahead. If you are at work during lunchtime, your choices are either taking a packed lunch or eating out. For those eating out, a word of caution – remember to steer well away from fried food, which is usually cooked in bad fats, also known as trans fats, hydrogenated oils, or vegetable oils. Fast food places love to use these because they are cheap. Trust me, sooner or later those motherfatters will mess you up.

Whenever you find yourself eating out, take just a second to look around at all the other folks frequenting your local food bar. If there are lots of vibrant, healthy looking people wearing spandex you should be good to go. If not, remember Farmer Fred? When all the animals at the same watering hole look sick, what does this tell you?

Before you find yourself sitting in a new restaurant take away some of the guesswork by Googling "Trip Adviser." This is a great resource for anyone travelling or on vacation. You'll find up-to-date reviews and reading other people's experiences is a sure way to gauge what to expect. You could also look for vegan/vegetarian/gluten free/paleo places.

THE SIX P RULE

For some of us, eating out can be a luxury. If your choices are eating out or paying the rent on time, then a packed lunch is not only a great way to save money, it also helps you have more control over what you put into your mouth. The trick to making this work is, once again, preparation. Remember the rule of Ps. Proper-planning-prevents-piss-poor-performance. Leaving everything until the last minute makes for a hungry, stressful day. A packed lunch is always best done the night before and then left in the fridge for morning.

Again, I'm not trying to win any medals for cooking here, but I am aware that there is a new generation that may not be used to preparing their own food. The whole idea of this chapter is to get them through to dinner without having to rely on any form of fast food. For those of us caught in a bind, the ideas offered here are quick and inexpensive.

There are a million and one great cookbooks out there and I'll be recommending one of them as we move through this chapter. But when I'm out and about, here are just a few simple ideas that I use. Are they perfect? Nope, like most people, I'm sometimes caught in less than optimal circumstances and just have to do the best I can. But it is possible to pack a lunch without resorting to sandwiches or grains. This doesn't have to be anything fancy and dollar for dollar they are a better value than eating out.

This first part I call a "lazy salad" because it's so quick and easy to make. Great if you can afford to go all organic, but if not, don't sweat it – any salad has to be a better option than eating deep fried fast food, am I right?

The night before, pick up a boxed mixed salad and toss some of it into some kind of Tupperware box along with some thinly sliced root vegetables like carrots, celery, broccoli, onion etc. If your local store has them, throw in a handful of freshly sprouted broccoli seeds and some olives (which are loaded with good fat). Bonus points if you can source these locally. Easy now with the condiments – instead, sprinkle a little apple cider vinegar, sea salt, and MCT oil if you have some over the salad and just for good measure you can even add a little turmeric.

Tip – To make life easier, buy a $1 plastic spray bottle, remove the spray section and screw it directly onto the top of your vinegar bottle. It works like a charm and is perfect for evenly applying vinegar to salads.

So far we have invested maybe five minutes of the day preparing this. Keep coming, we are almost there. For protein you could try adding in any leftovers from the night before. If you do okay with eggs, then two boiled eggs should help keep you going. If you really are pressed for time, try sardines direct from the can. Hey, sardines have enough selenium to counter any mercury found in the sea. And they are a quick, easy, and good source of good fats. They are also a healthier option than eating fast food for lunch.

If you really want to be ahead of the game you can take a hot thermos flask filled with homemade soup. Homemade soup is super easy to make and it's something I cover in the next chapter. Note, so far none of these ideas have included gluten. Keep in mind when we remove gluten in the form of bread and pasta etc. we also remove an element of fiber. Some of us may need more fiber than others to help keep our bowel movements regular, again we are all unique. Fortunately, there are other ways of getting fiber without piling bread on your plate.

If you can tolerate it, one way is to eat more brown rice which, once cooked, can later be eaten cold. Brown rice has far more fiber than white rice. Yup, I already know about the higher arsenic content of brown rice, but remember these are your do-or-die tips for folks who may be new to preparing their own food. And these tips are a step up from eating out. Fiber is important for healthy gut bacteria because it serves as a pre-biotic. Whenever you cook rice, try adding a little pasture-raised butter. Despite what they tell you, this is a form of good fat and it will help keep hunger at bay.

For dessert, let's not go too crazy with the fruit. Maybe go with berries or, to keep things interesting, peel and slice a Granny Smith apple. Typically, Granny Smith apples have less sugar than most of those new hybrid apples. Feel free to add a squirt of lemon juice directly onto the sliced apple to stop it from going brown (nope, no need to genetically modify it).

Many people like to pack a banana for lunch, but be aware that they can be pretty high in sugar so, as always, moderation is key. I'm sure we have all heard that bananas are a good source of potassium but if it's potassium you are after you could also go avocado instead. Avocado ticks the good fat, good fiber box and it's lower in sugar than a banana. To boost the fat content of these desserts try whisking them up with cream of coconut – this usually comes in a can, but hey, we are in survival mode here so it all counts and adding berries to it makes it okay.

If you find yourself getting hungry between meals, try nibbling on sliced coconut or a small piece of ginger to tame that snack attack. Ginger can be peeled quickly by using the back of a spoon, try it for yourself and see. Ginger has more health benefits than you or I can shake a hairy stick at and it's a great way to stop rewarding yourself with all those unhealthy snacks.

Your absolute number one best option for a drink is always going to be natural spring water. Forget all those "healthy" fruit juices (unless you are vegetable juicing of course). Without the fiber, fruits are simply liquid sugar in a carton. If you have a problem quitting soda, don't shoot yourself in the foot by going sugar free. Additives used in those sugar free drinks are not your friend. If you really need that fizzy-fix you could try switching to kombucha provided you aren't dealing with an ongoing candida issue. Even then I suspect this is a much better option than soda. You can find kombucha in most health food stores and in the long run it's also better for you than all those crash and burn high caffeine energy drinks.

Tip – Wherever you live in the world you can usually find a freshwater spring that's close to you by clicking on your address at "findaspring.com." It always pays to test any new water source, however, and this is easy to do with a quick Google search.

KIDS

Kids are funny – I should know, I used to be one. Ask any kid if they would like some sliced up coconut with cucumber and carrots dipped in hummus and they will inevitably say no. Now, if you pay close attention you will notice that kids spend an inordinate amount of their time hanging off the fridge door complaining there is nothing to eat. Use this to your advantage.

Kids are visual; if foods are cut up and arranged in bold colors right in front of them, they will be more tempted to try them. Inside the fridge, strategically place several open containers of the most random healthy things you can think of and set them at kids' eye level. You can add to the visual by buying small colorful berry bowls for about a buck a piece.

Kids also like to see how far they can push you. If that's how your crew rolls, then you can even try a little reverse phycology. First, make the containers of cut of vegetables look attractive and then tell your kids not to eat them. It may also help to have some form of healthy dip on hand too. Once it's in front of them, sooner or later they will eat it – even if it's only to tell you how gross it is. I know right, getting a kid to eat healthy can be like negotiating with a terrorist.

To save on waste, don't use big containers. It could be just a few well-placed bowls that might include any of the following: sliced olives, cut ginger, purple cabbage, sliced coconut, chopped broccoli, sliced carrots, cucumber, quartered or sliced boiled egg, sugar snap peas, thinly sliced celery, radishes, sprouts, yada, yada, yada. Obviously I'm just making a few suggestions and I'm not saying to put all of these out in one day. Try rotating them and see what works best for you. Kids are notoriously fickle eaters. It's not uncommon for them to also develop a bad habit of eating potato chips. Ideally we want to wean them off chips altogether, but for now let's not initiate a full blown mutiny. If this is you, try buying only plain chips. Make no mistake, plain flavored chips still have undesirable things in them but the idea is that during the transition time, kids will eat fewer of them.

Whatever you try, it helps to use a little imagination. But always remember to go easy on the fruit, especially when it's out of season. If this all seems like work, remember this is easier than being held hostage to cook meals throughout the day – and so far it's also been a pretty easy day for the dishwasher. Now you dunnit it.

Is it me, or is the dishwasher the only home appliance we make excuses for? Ask yourself if you are really just "rinsing" those dirty dishes before putting them in the dishwasher or have we all been hoodwinked into doing the job we've paid the dishwasher manufacturers to do?

Think about it, what if suddenly we had to rinse all our dirty socks before we put them in the washing machine? Or we had to partially iron our clothes before asking the iron to step up and do its job. I know, right? People would be in the streets rioting with pitchforks – and rightly so.

We have the technology to put a robot on Mars and yet we still have to "rinse" dirty dishes before we dare put them in the dishwasher.

Really? I'm telling you, those damned dishwasher sales men are laughing all the way to the bank. Ask yourself, when was the last time you saw a homeless dishwasher salesman? No, you never have because they are all too busy driving around in expensive sports cars and smoking oversized, hand-rolled Cuban cigars. But I digress.

SPROUTING

Imagine having a vegetable garden that produces clean nutrition year round with no weeding, no back breaking digging, no bugs, no green thumb necessary, no greenhouse, and not even any soil. And now imagine that the crops from this garden have a higher nutritional content than any whole food found in the supermarket! Better still, imagine that this crop can be grown within days on your kitchen counter. It's incredibly cost effective and simple to do.

Sprouts are something you can include in your lunchtime meals and sprouting involves very little in the way of materials. It's so easy to do a child can do it – you catching my drift? Sprouting is a great way to get them to eat their healthy greens. This becomes easier and more fun when kids get to experiment with sprouting and see things sprout as quickly as overnight. Sprouted seeds are packed with nutrients and live enzymes. For sensitive individuals, sprouts can be a superior way to get your key nutrients rather than taking synthetic vitamins.

There really isn't too much to sprouting. Simply buy some sprouting seeds online or locally and allow them to soak in a glass jar. Usually the soaking period is twelve hours. Keep rinsing them off until they sprout. During sprouting, it's obviously important to keep everything clean. The key here is to regularly rinse the sprouted seeds to make sure they don't get any mold on them – but beyond that, there isn't much to do. If you are just starting out, try starting with some of the larger seeds, it's just easier all round. For the first couple of times,

DON'T sprout more than a tablespoonful, this is a project you should grow into (yup, meant that pun).

Here's a simple formula for sprouting:

- Buy (LARGE) seeds from a local store or a sprouting company online
- Soak the seeds
- Pour the seeds into a strainer
- Rinse every couple of hours
- Watch for tails to sprout from the seeds
- Keep rinsing to stop them from drying out
- Always check for mold

Sprouting is good to try because:

- Anyone can do it
- It adds vital nutrients to the body
- It's inexpensive
- It doesn't involve a lot of time
- You don't need a big garden
- Sprouting even can even be done in a small apartment, caravan, or RV

There are lots of places to buy the sprouting seeds; you can buy them online or even at your local supermarket. Sproutpeople.org is an online supplier that offers decent products along with more detailed information and equipment if you need it. The bulk of the information is given freely on their site.

If your system is fragile or just out of balance, sprouting can be a good way to get key nutrients into your body. Learning about nutrient-dense foods, superfoods, sprouts, and juicing is a lot easier to do than learning about supplements, and can be a lot less problematic.

KICKING OLD HABITS

Whenever we change the way we eat, simple plans tend to work better than complicated ones, and no plan will work if you don't understand it. The bigger challenge is to get you to let go of old habits. I have a friend – let's call him Tom – who once asked me if I knew of a quick fix to help with his abdominal pain. It had developed over the past few months and had become a real problem whenever he ate salt and vinegar chips.

At considerable cost, his doctor had already performed an esophagogastroduodenoscopy (EGD) test to examine the lining of the esophagus, stomach, and first part of the small intestine with a camera. Nothing obvious was discovered and Tylenol was prescribed for the pain.

Over the next fifteen minutes, Tom continued to divulge the full symptoms of his stomach which now included nausea from taking the Tylenol. Finally, he stopped talking long enough to ask me what I thought. After a moment of deep thought I said that a solution was indeed available to him as the technician operating the expensive camera inside his body had missed something of critical importance.

Eagerly he listened as I motioned with my hand for him to come a little closer. As he leaned in to better hear what I had to say I gently whispered in his ear … "Tom, just stop eating the chips."

A month or so passed and not a single chip passed his lips, and as if by sorcery his problem went away and never came back! Later it was declared by his doctor that his gut pain had gone into a form of spontaneous remission. Maybe the reason Tom succeeded was simply because he'd implemented that simple change.

Again, if this is all new to you, don't panic. A good rule of thumb is to simply fill 50% of every plate you serve yourself with green leafy vegetables. Do this one thing and you will be ahead of the pack.

I fully appreciate that sometimes all this can be a little difficult to understand, which is why I've been so keen to recommend several blogs along the way. To be fair, there simply isn't room to list all the good ones I've taken information from over the years and it's been a real internal struggle for me to have to leave some of them out.

The ones I'm recommending here are snapshots that represent so many others. This next one comes from a lady who makes highly informative videos covering a wide range of topics. Check her out in today's homework.

What did we learn from this chapter?

Thinking about meals ahead of time is the key to your success. Having something quick and easy that's prepared ahead of time can stop a snack attack in its tracks. If you wait until you are hungry before figuring out what snacks you are going to eat, then everything becomes hard.

Homework: Check out montrealhealthygirl.com, or search for her videos on YouTube. Brittany has an extensive understanding of the healing process and she always manages to pack a few gems into her videos. She has a genuine passion for helping people, which is very apparent and oozes through in her highly informative videos. Link: https://www.youtube.com/watch?v=dWO5ufhPLc4

Chapter 17

WHAT THE HELL DO I EAT FOR DINNER?

Anything you decide to cook for dinner is only going to be as good as the ingredients you use. Finding local produce is my preferred option, but should supply be thin on the ground, don't panic because it's not your only option. If you know where to find it, organic produce can be delivered directly to you. And often a simple Google search will give you options in your area. These days you can even get grass-fed meat delivered direct to your door. Meat arrives fresh, sealed, and frozen via the miracle of dry ice. I've occasionally used Butcher box.com; the meat is quality and they ship for free. Once you have your materials the next step is to find a way to save on time.

Cooking a healthy meal from scratch can be time consuming which is why a pressure cooker is a useful addition to any kitchen. Pressure cookers typically cook a meal 70% faster than regular cookers. Pressure cookers are also a good way to reduce the lectin content of certain foods, which is something we covered earlier. If you have never used a pressure cooker you are in for a pleasant surprise.

OMG, THE NO PRESSURE, PRESSURE COOKER

When time is limited there can be a lot of pressure surrounding mealtimes, so here's a clever idea that's gives you control of your kitchen. Hear me out on this one because even though pressure cookers have been around for a long time, they recently went all electric. This not only made things safer, it also made cooking a whole lot easier and faster. If you only take away one tip from this chapter, then please let it be this: Google the Instant Pot. You can literally throw food in an Instant Pot, walk away, and come back to a hot meal in half the time! The Instant Pot has revolutionized cooking and for those who are culinarily challenged like me, cooking with an Instant

Pot is a game changer. The Instant Pot was the first kitchen appliance to ever go viral, and with no advertising it quickly sold out.

It's fair to say that if my wife ever decided to run off with my best friend (a) I'd sure miss him and (b) this is probably how I'd feed myself until he came to his senses.

There is an entire Instant Pot community on Facebook. I like to refer to them as potheads. Potheads offer lots of helpful recipes to get you started and the Instant Pot also comes with its own helpful cookbook. The one I have in my kitchen is sold on Amazon for around $99. It offers good value for the money because it doubles as a slow cooker with the added benefit of using a stainless steel pot. It's a win/win. As with any product I recommend, my primary affiliation is always with you. With that in mind, I have refrained from putting in a direct link – that way you know I am recommending this product because it works rather than trying to profit from any kind of affiliated kick back.

REGULAR SLOW COOKER

Even without a pressure cooker, another option is to use a good old regular slow cooker. While this option isn't quite as rock and roll as the Instant Pot, slow cookers are generally less expensive to buy and a useful tool to help get a hot meal on the table.

For those who are used to eating out of a can, here's a super easy way to make homemade chicken soup (trust me, I'm no cook and even I struggle to get this one wrong). Preparing this meal takes maybe ten minutes. Do it in the morning and you always have a healthy hot meal to come home to. This style of cooking is real back-to-basics and pretty hard to mess up. You can obviously leave out anything that you are sensitive to.

For this example, simply place a whole chicken (preferably free range, local, or organic) into a slow cooker or large cooking type stock pot. Add enough water to cover the chicken, chop up and add a couple of onions and some vegetables. These can by anything; maybe throw in some carrots, broccoli, celery, mushrooms, cabbage, potatoes, garlic etc.

Add a teaspoon of Himalayan salt and turn it up high to get it cooking and then let simmer with the bones still in for a good few hours. If you have a low enough setting you can even let it simmer overnight, which adds to the flavor. As long as you are happy that the chicken is cooked you can let it simmer for as little or as long as you like. That's it! Obviously remove all bones before serving. The more times you make this meal the easier it gets. Sometimes I'll add a little turmeric and ginger. It's really not an exact science, just practice, eat, and repeat.

Tip – You can also add a tablespoon of apple cider vinegar to the soup as it simmers. This will help leech more minerals out of the bones. Minerals are what most of us are deficient in. Cooking with pasture-raised, wild caught, and organic meats generally increases the mineral count.

Waiting until you are hungry to figure out what's for dinner is a sure recipe for frustration. Planning ahead is the key to a successful outcome. The chicken soup is a cost-effective meal that typically feeds a family of four twice over. It's the opposite of a microwave meal and your Roman ancestors probably made a similar version as they marched across Europe bossing people about.

BONE BROTH

Bone broths are a super healthy option and are easy to make. Typically, bone broth is made using the bones of pasture-raised beef, lamb, pork, chicken, or even the heads from wild caught fish. Bone broth is best left simmering for a minimum of eight hours – but to get the most minerals out of bones, longer is better. Beef bones can cook for up to forty-eight hours. To help flood the broth with minerals, add vinegar to the water. While the bone broth simmers, you can also add your favorite herbs or vegetables to help make the taste more palatable. Once cooked, either sip on the liquid or use it as gravy poured over meals. You can even freeze any leftovers to give flavor to a later dish. Although you can certainly cook a bone broth on the stove top using a regular large pan, I find it easier to leave it in a slow cooker.

Tip – Given that minerals are essential for the absorption of vitamins, think of bone broth as a daily multi-mineral alternative. Bone broths are a great way to safely increase mineral intake, this can be a particularly useful way for sensitive individuals to get their minerals. It's worth noting that without minerals, vitamins cannot be absorbed properly.

The amount of minerals found in bone broth is largely dependent on the quality of the bones. Finding bones from grass- or pasture-raised animals in your area is easy to do with a quick Google search.

Bone broth is a solid staple of the paleo diet because it contains an abundance of the amino acids arginine, glycine, glutamine, and proline. All of these amino acids have powerful healing properties, especially for the lining of the gut. Some digestive issues can be helped with a bone broth fast; some believe a three-day bone broth fast can help heal the damaged lining of the gut. Bone broth can help alleviate joint pain and boost your immune system. Bone broth is collagen-rich and collagen is known to tighten the skin and even make your hair shiny.

If you don't have the time to make bone broth for yourself, Dr. Axe has an instant powdered bone broth that literally takes 5 minutes to make.

Recommended reading – The Keto Diet by Leanne Vogel. I'm currently halfway through reading this and I can tell it's going to be one of my go-to books. It's beautifully designed, well written, and all her recipes are easy to follow.

What did we learn from this chapter?

Cooking at home gives you greater control over what you eat. This is helpful for anyone with food sensitivities. Bone broths come loaded with minerals and amino acids which can help heal the gut.

Homework: to help keep this information balanced, here's a wonderful short video by Christa Orecchio. Christa always puts out clear, easy to understand information which is sure to put a smile on your face. Check out the link below.

https://thewholejourney.com/is-a-ketogenic-diet-good-or-bad/

Chapter 18

FREESTYLING

One of the problems with blindly taking supplements is that so many health problems today link back to an immune system that's been spooked. With over a hundred autoimmune conditions to choose from, it's plausible that many patients are undiagnosed or even misdiagnosed. This is important because many supplements are capable of tipping the Th1 Th2 balance too far in one direction. If you have been down the pill-popping road and felt worse for it, then perhaps consider autoimmunity as an option.

There are a lot of variables surrounding supplementation and they can at times be incalculable. You may recall that we first talked about this back in Chapter 13. What works well for one person might not bring the same results in another.

While there could be many reasons for such differences, I suspect that in illness, the liver and kidneys are usually pulling a double shift and, as you can imagine, taxing an already overloaded system with handfuls of supplements rarely bodes well. Keep in mind that the liver performs a wide range of bodily functions; some estimates suggest that the liver is involved in more than 500 hundred different functions! It's imperative we show it some respect.

Still, there are times when genuine deficiencies need to be addressed in the body and that, my friend, is the aim of this chapter! The fact that this subject is so late in the book highlights my reluctance to lead you down a pill-popping path. The problem is that many of us have become quick to think of pill-popping as an effective solution. It is not.

So why do we need supplements?

In a perfect world we wouldn't need them at all and no doubt there was a time when we could have gotten all our vitamins and minerals from the foods we ate. If your body could talk to you, this would be the preferable way. However, modern farming practices are quick to bring crops to market and slow to allow the soil time to recover. This really means that anyone eating standard supermarket food will at some point usually need to plug a few nutrient gaps.

So let's back up and ask how our early ancestors managed to survive without pockets full of pills? The short answer is right under your feet. Today, as never before, our soils are in a state of exhaustion.

To compensate for their lack of trace minerals, farmers have learned to prop up the soil with chemical additives. Doing this only serves to compound the problem because it causes an imbalance of trace minerals and disrupts the life cycle of important microorganisms found in the soil.

SOIL

We should first think of soil as a bank account. If you take too much out, you have to deposit some back in or the soil simply becomes bankrupt – and this is where we are today. Our ancestors had the good sense to rotate crops and give the soil time to recover. Today we feed our crops harsh chemicals and fertilizers in an attempt to force them grow quicker. Make no mistake, the result is more profitable crops for the farmer, but for your body's cells, those missing minerals soon add up to have a negative effect on your health.

Side by side, crops grown this way may look the same, but vegetables absorb these important trace minerals through their roots – which you then eat. Your trillions of tiny cells require a wide range of trace minerals to keep your body running optimally.

Let's be clear, whenever food is grown for profit, it arrives on your kitchen table devoid of important minerals. When the soil becomes mineral deficient you become mineral deficient!

Whatever minerals were found in farm soil 100, fifty or even twenty-five years ago are almost certainly not found in the soil today. Today, commercially grown, nutrient deficient crops are really imposters of the real thing. They may look the same as regular crops, but they are weaker than their clean cousins and as such are more susceptible to bug infestations. Man's solution? Spray the crops with more poisons! I know, right? You couldn't make this stuff up.

Think of it this way:

> Man owes his existence to a six-inch layer of topsoil—
> and the fact that it rains.
> – Anonymous

Our great grandparents had a solution to solve this mineral depletion and it wasn't at all complicated. They knew that if they placed old food scraps in a small garden pile, the scraps would gradually decompose. This decomposed matter could then be added back into the soil as compost creating a perfect cycle. A compost pile costs zero money to build and yet it's incredibly beneficial to the soil. This process is really nothing more than putting the nutrients back into the soil the old fashioned way.

Many of our small, local farmers today still work this way, and as I mentioned earlier, many of these small farmers may or may not have the organic seal and that's okay too. For my money, knowing a small farmer who understands soil by name is of equal importance.

The answer to nutrient-poor foods that society has come up with is to sell you synthetic multivitamins. Often these types of low-end vitamins are sold in large discount stores and do more harm than good. Quality is key with any supplement, and there is some merit to occasionally taking a food-based multivitamin, but even this can have drawbacks.

Given that we are each unique it can be a real challenge to find a single pill to fit all our needs. Running parallel with this problem is the current upsurge in thyroid and autoimmune diseases and the fact that many of the ingredients in the pills can even make you feel worse. So what's the answer? First, know that you simply cannot supplement your way out of a bad diet and with a good diet most people don't need supplements. Second, perhaps adopt a more targeted approach to occasionally using supplements. When we are trying to hit a nutritional target, we could think of the standard multivitamin as a shotgun approach, i.e., as hitting a broad number of targets. A more targeted approach would be like using a sniper rifle with a telescopic lens.

The easy way to ensure your food has the vital minerals you need is to bring this full circle and grow some of your own food. This is something you can do even with a single raised bed measuring just 4ft x 8ft. As any simple soil test demonstrates, foods grown in nutrient dense soils have more minerals. When you run the cost side by side, home grown food simply outperforms all other options. As soon as I am settled again, planting a garden will be my number one priority. For now, I'm still trying to adjust to my new living environment and like millions of others my diet has become less than ideal.

With that in mind, here are some of the supplements I occasionally take myself and why. Unless you know why you are taking a supplement, then really you have no business putting it in your mouth. I also make a point of tracking everything I take in a day planner to monitor results. I strongly urge you to do the same. Keeping your notes simple makes this process so much easier to do.

Over the years I've tried literally hundreds of different supplements. And some of them worked better than others. For me, rather than being brand loyal or tied to any one supplement long term, I respond better when I switch it up from time to time. At the moment I am working with "Black-Seed oil," and enjoying the many benefits of this all round tonic (despite the taste). When I feel it's positive effects weaning, I'll move onto something else. I refer to this style of supplementing as "freestyling."

As long as I feel a benefit from taking a supplement I'll stick with it, but as soon as I feel the benefits begin to plateau, I'll drop it like a hot potato and rotate to the next supplement. At some point I'll eventually cycle back around to the same supplement. This style of rotating my supplements seems to works for me, perhaps because over time I'm covering more bases, or perhaps because I've simply become better at trusting my own intuition. Unfortunately, the downside of this means I'm sometimes left with a graveyard of half-used supplement bottles.

But remember, although there are many beneficial supplements on the market, the least complicated route is to get the lion's share of your minerals and vitamins from clean nutrition, bone broths, foods grown in nutrient dense soils, and pasture-raised meats. All these are much easier to get right than are supplements.

As our time is now quickly running out, I guess I'm forced to narrow this down a little. Obviously, all minerals and vitamins play an important role in the body but if I were about to be stranded on a desert island I would hope to have with me the following: a good probiotic, magnesium, a form of krill oil, and good old vitamin C. If you are wondering why I didn't mention the all-important vitamin D it's because on this desert island I'd imagine there would be plenty of sunshine – so perhaps I'll go with a B complex instead.

Trying to narrow so many supplements down to just five is a difficult challenge because there are so many other compounds that play an important role in good health. Hence the reason I tend to "cycle" often which typically means I'm hitting more bases over time. Is this a perfect system? Nope, but to be honest, when it comes to taking supplements I've yet to see a system that is. Either way, let's first take a look at probiotics.

PROBIOTICS help increase the amount of good bacteria found inside the gut and are typically taken orally. It's debatable, but for my money I highly rate probiotic supplements simply because it's estimated that the bacteria in your body outnumber your cells by about ten to one. That could be as many as 100 trillion bacteria living inside you! If you think about it, you are actually more bacteria than you are human. I know, right? All that antibacterial soap is slowly killing you!

Typically, the majority of these bacteria live in the intestinal system which we now know is heavily involved with the immune system and even serotonin production. Given the significance of this, it's important to optimize the health of the bacteria in the gut in any way we can and probiotic supplementation is one way. There is some debate surrounding which probiotics work best, but it really doesn't matter how good your probiotic is if the bad bacteria in your gut are being fed excessive amounts of sugar.

Keep in mind there are things that nourish the good bacteria and there are things that can accelerate the growth of bad bacteria. One of the fastest ways to upset this balance is to take antibiotics. Obviously there are times when this is unavoidable which makes the topic of probiotics all the more valid because probiotics help repopulate the gut bacteria. It's probably worth mentioning that approximately 70% of all the antibiotics being manufactured today are used in the food supply. I know, right? Ever wonder what happens when we eat the animal that eats antibiotics?

Where we choose to buy the foods we eat will have a profound effect on the delicate balance of good and bad bacteria in our gut. One of the most effective ways to help suppress the bad bacteria is to limit your sugar intake. Sugar feeds bad bacteria and let's not forget that fruit, and fruit juices in particular, are also loaded with sugar – some more than others.

On the flip side, clean, whole vegetables help feed the good bacteria. The fiber in these foods can be thought of as pre-biotics. You can also eat foods that are high in natural probiotics such as fermented vegetables like sauerkraut, kimchi, and certain pickled vegetables – preferably organic when possible because most non-organic produce is sprayed with harsh chemicals that may affect those trillions of good bacteria that live inside you.

Be aware that store-bought yogurt and kefir is typically loaded with sugars and additives despite what the marketing on the label says. Also, if your water is chlorinated it's going to affect your good bacteria. Knowing that our tiny gut bugs make up 90% of who we are, some estimates suggest those tiny gut bugs outnumber our cells by 10 to 1. Perhaps we should be showing them a little more respect. Dump the junk water and go with natural spring water whenever possible.

Whenever you make bold moves to change the good bugs in your stomach it's best to start small and go slow. An ideal starting point is to gradually introduce fermented foods into your diet, especially if you are dealing with candida. When it comes to supplementing with probiotics some are best taken on an empty stomach and others require food, so always read the label. There are lots of good probiotics on the market. Given that we are all so different a little trial and error can be expected. When you hit the right probiotic you may feel your overall mood improves, the time to switch is when that feeling plateaus.

As a rule of thumb, try to steer clear of bargain priced probiotics. In my opinion you are better off paying a little extra and getting a quality probiotic. Here are three suggestions, but there are plenty of other good probiotics on the market. Prescript-Assist sells a probiotic that is made up of SBOs (soil based organisms). Whenever I look to switch things around a little, I also seem to do well with a probiotic made by Elixa Probiotic, although at the time of writing they are currently sold out in the U.S.

Dr. Mercola also sells a good probiotic as does Standard Process which is their prosynbiotic probiotic. These aren't the only four options out there; I'm just trying to save you a little time. Ultimately it's important to find one that works for you.

MAGNESIUM makes it to the list not because it's an essential mineral but because it covers so many bases. From head to toe magnesium is involved in more than 300 metabolic reactions. It can help with everything from normalizing blood pressure to keeping a steady heart rhythm. A lack of magnesium can play a key role in anxiety and fatigue and it may surprise some to know that magnesium even plays a key role in the skeletal system. For sure, it's just as important to the health of your bones as calcium is. Magnesium also made it to the list because a deficiency can be caused as a result of parasitic infection, candida overgrowth, or as a result of a poor diet such as the Standard American Diet. However, before you rush out to add it to your routine you should know there is a little more to magnesium supplementation than meets the eye.

Magnesium is not easily absorbed in pill form. Its ability to be utilized in the body is co-dependent on several other compounds such as calcium and vitamins D and K2. This tight group is commonly found together in certain foods such as spinach and other dark leafy greens, also in fish in the form of mackerel – hence the reason I keep harping that plate in front of you contain 50% dark green leafy veggies and that diet is so important.

Also, keep in mind there are nine common types of magnesium, all of which differ slightly in the benefits they offer. Perhaps this is another reason I find it helpful to switch things around from time to time. If you are just starting out, try applying magnesium transdermally, which simply means applying it to the skin. Doing it this way helps with absorption issues. Transdermal magnesium can be bought in lotion form and is ideal for sensitive individuals or children. Ancient Minerals is a decent enough product and a simple Google search will take you to it.

Another way to load magnesium is by adding magnesium bath salts to your bath and soaking in them. Ideally, steer clear of any product with added perfume in the ingredients. Ultimately, let yourself be guided by how each makes you feel. For those attempting oral supplementation, it may prove helpful to try alternating with either magnesium citrate or magnesium orotate. If you find yourself drawn to cycling either of these forms, always take them in sensible moderation rather than trying too much all at once.

KRILL OIL is loaded with the omega-3 polyunsaturated fatty acids DHA (docosahexaenoic) and EPA (eicosapentaenoic acid). Both of these help keep the brain firing on all four cylinders. Krill oil is unique because unlike regular fish oils it can be absorbed directly by the brain with very little processing. It may also help support better concentration, memory, and learning. Krill oil also has more antioxidants than regular fish oil and is generally considered safer

because of its lower levels of contaminants such as mercury. Mercury can be a problem, especially in tuna, marlin, and swordfish.
Krill oil also contains astaxanthin which can be helpful to the eyes. Given that the eyes have a high density of mitochondria, some reports suggest astaxanthin helps protect mitochondria from oxidative stress. Just for good measure, krill oil is thought to support a healthy heart, the brain, and the nervous system as well as keep cholesterol and blood lipids in the normal range. It also helps maintain healthy blood sugar levels, keeps joints healthy, supports liver function, and even supports the immune system.

VITAMIN C is a water-soluble vitamin, which means your body doesn't store it. Humans do not have the ability to make vitamin C as many animals do, which means you need to consume it via your diet. This is one reason vitamin C made it to the list but also because it covers so many bases.

Vitamin C is my go-to supplement whenever I feel a cold coming on, but the benefits of vitamin C can be used to treat a much wider range of health problems. It's also known to be useful in wound healing and skin health. It can be used to treat joint and muscle problems and it plays a role in a healthy heart. Yup, you heard me right on that last one.

When it comes to the heart, vitamin C is right up there with healthy exercise. Vitamin C is a powerful antioxidant, known to block some of the damage caused by DNA-damaging free radicals. Over time, free radical damage may accelerate aging and contribute to the development of heart disease. Vitamin C also benefits the eyes and is thought to lower your risk of cataracts. Vitamin C supports the immune system and is important for respiratory health. Larger doses can be useful for allergies and asthma due to its antioxidant and anti-inflammatory effect.

The brain and nervous system also have a need for vitamin C. Some sources suggest deficiencies can lead to a degeneration of the nervous system with possible links to neurological based diseases such as ALS, Parkinson's, and Alzheimer's. Vitamin C is needed to help keep the tissue in the digestive tract healthy and has been shown to be useful for stomach ulcers, gastritis, and H. Pylori, which is a bacterium known to cause chronic inflammation/infection in the stomach and duodenum.

The recommended daily allowance (RDA) for vitamin C has been established at 40 to 60 mg per day although some might suggest this is on the low end. According to Nobel Prize winning scientist Linus Pauling, elevated doses of vitamin C may have a role to play in the fight against cancer. Pauling spent his life advocating amounts of 1,000 mg or even higher until he died at the age of ninety-three. High doses of Vitamin C are sometimes administered by IV.

Most take Vitamin C orally. The brand I personally use is sold by Beyond-Health. It's a little pricey but compared to buying all those cold and flu remedies from the pharmacy it evens out in the long run. An ounce of prevention is always better than a pound of cure. This brand of vitamin C is a buffered powder and contains trace amounts of potassium, calcium magnesium, and zinc.

You can also increase your vitamin C level by squeezing a fresh lemon or lime into water and drinking it. It might surprise some to know that red peppers are high in vitamin C and compared to oranges they obviously have less sugar. For anyone with an iron deficiency, pairing Vitamin C with iron has been shown to improve absorption, although another option would be to eat more beef liver. Pairing Vitamin C with the amino acid N-acetylcysteine (NAC) is an inexpensive way to help the body build glutathione, which is considered the body's master antioxidant.

Another option to increase glutathione is to use a liposomal glutathione supplement which helps the glutathione be better absorbed through the GI tract. If you can afford it, a more efficient way to increase glutathione is by IV, although this option is not only more expensive it also requires a qualified doctor to be in the loop. Glutathione administered via an IV has been shown to be helpful in the fight against Parkinson's disease. But I digress.

Not all B-COMPLEX supplements are made equal and again you are better off steering well clear of bargain basement supplements. A whole foods-based B-complex is the preferred way to go and there are plenty of good ones on the market. B vitamins play an important role in keeping the body energized throughout the day as well as helping convert our food into fuel. The idea of taking a good quality B-complex is that it has eight B vitamins added which include, B1, B2, B3, B5, B6, B7, B9 and sometimes B12.

B12 is a big one as it does so much in the body. It can also be purchased on its own. A B12 deficiency can sometimes leave a person feeling tired or unfocused and can also sometimes be coupled with a dizzy feeling or even heart palpitations. With so many overlapping symptoms, getting an accurate diagnosis can be particularly problematic. Typically, a B12 deficiency is measured based on the serum vitamin B12 levels within the blood. As we all know, standard blood tests are not infallible and there are times when some patients will fall through the cracks. A more precise screening might be one that checks for high homocysteine levels. Unfortunately, this test is usually only given to patients who have a known case of anemia or heart disease-related symptoms.

Sometimes doing things the old school way by cross-checking a list of symptoms can prove just as helpful. Things to be on the lookout for might include an inability to concentrate, chronic fatigue, muscle weakness, joint pain, shortness of breath, dizziness, poor memory, heart palpitations, bleeding gums, a poor appetite, digestive problems, and even mood changes such as depression and anxiety. While there could be any number of reasons for the above symptoms, it's important to note that a deficiency in B12 is more likely to occur in someone who has absorption issues in the gut (hello again cheeky-leaky). Some vegans may also lean toward a B12 deficiency. The elderly are particularly prone to B12 deficiency and for anyone with a relative showing signs of early dementia, adding a B-complex supplement will prove beneficial. Foods high in B12 are beef, chicken, liver, and fish such as wild caught salmon, herring, mackerel, and sardines.

When supplementing, keep in mind that the body strives to remain in balance and sometimes this challenge is best tackled with herbs. Herbs have been used in medicine since the beginning of time and some are far more potent than others. It's worth noting that herbs such as Echinacea, astragalus, olive leaf, cat's claw, elderberry, and goldenseal all have the potential to crank up the immune system.

While this may be the desired effect for many, for the autoimmune patient this can be a double-edged sword. However, all is not lost. There is a subcategory of herbs known as adaptogenic herbs. Put simply, these herbs help the body adapt. Rather than stimulate, they are known to soothe the immune system, hence the name adaptogenic. For some, adaptogens may prove to be the missing link.

ADAPTOGENS

When used in conjunction with a clean diet, think of adaptogenic herbs as a natural substance which assist the body in adapting to stress and to help bring a normalizing effect upon bodily processes. Adaptogens are highly versatile which can be especially useful when trying to balance out either Th1 or Th2 dominance of the immune system.

Adaptogens can help increase the body's resistance to mental, physical, and environmental stress, although results will be hindered if the original stressor (i.e. food allergy) remains a constant. We briefly mentioned Cordyceps earlier which are not adaptogens in the classic sense, but they do have adaptogenic qualities, hence they get a quick mentioned again here.

What follows is a very basic summary of some widely used adaptogens. If this is all new to you, try to find an experienced herbalist to work with.

Ashwagandha has been used in Ayurvedic medicine for over 2000 years. Its immuno-modulating effects help the body adapt to stress. It can also be helpful in treating anxiety.

Ginseng is probably one of the more well-used adaptogens among herbalists. Asian ginseng is used most often because it is the most potent of the ginseng family. Studies show that Asian ginseng has great antioxidant effects, as well as helping your body adapt to stress. In some people it can be helpful in lowering blood pressure.

I've put Chaste Tree Berry (vitex agnus-castus) on the list especially for the ladies. Chase tree mimics the master hormone, progesterone. So what does that mean? Well for starters, better balanced hormones =less stress, less PMS, and less difficulty transitioning into menopause! Although it may take up to eight weeks to feel the full effect, Chaste Tree can be a total game changer for many women. Give it time and it may just be your silver bullet.

Holy Basil helps fight fatigue and stabilize your immune system. It can also be used to regulate blood sugar and hormone levels.

Rhodiola is another potent adaptogen that has had many research studies done on it. Rhodiola helps the body adapt to stress-induced mental and physical fatigue. Studies found that Rhodiola restores normal patterns of eating and sleeping after long-term stress. It also helps combat mental and physical fatigue, protects against oxidative stress, heat stress, radiation, and exposure to toxic chemicals. Rhodiola also protects the heart and liver, increases use of oxygen, and improves memory.

Gynostemma (or jiaogulan, as it's sometimes called) is another adaptogenic herb and a potent health tonic made as a tea. In addition to helping balance the immune system, it also increases stamina and helps reduce stress. Gynostemma has a slightly woody taste which, given its health benefits, doesn't faze me in the slightest.

The 2nd HEALING TRIANGLE

Okay, I know the sands of time are quickly running out on us, so a more serious illness may call for a more a direct approach. So before we leave this section, I'd like to quickly mention the idea of a 2nd healing triangle. As mentioned earlier, your liver plays a key role in your recovery. If you are smart, treat your liver like your new BF and it will become a formidable ally to have on your team. Right now, even as we talk, your liver is busy doing everything it can to protect you from a daily assault of toxic chemicals. It's currently performing a wide range of tasks just to keep you alive. For this reason, the liver forms the first part of this triangle.

Hear this: every year we change the oil in our cars, perhaps you change your own oil or perhaps you pay someone to do it for you. Every time you take your car in for an oil change, did you ever stop and think about your liver? Occasionally it needs to be cleaned too.

There are many ways to do this and by now I hope you have a basic grasp on how to do this. If all else fails, find someone to help you the same way you would pay someone to change your oil. If money is tight, this book is full of people and places where you can find more answers. Earthclinic.com often has interesting information to offer.

Next, we should by now also know that sugar has become a thorn in the side of all humankind. It's everywhere and anywhere; it's plastered on billboards and even sold to our kids in schools. So much illness has its roots firmly planted in sugar. A reduction of sugar may prove helpful, but as we know sugar can be an additive. If you currently face a serious health challenge, simply reducing your known sugar intake may not be enough.

Fortunately, the second part of this triangle deals with this problem quite well. The ketogenic diet comes in many forms. Find a nutritionist who understands the importance of cutting sugar to a wellness level based on your individual needs. Starving the body of sugar is the second part of our triangle, but this doesn't mean you have to starve yourself. As we mentioned earlier, the body already knows how to burn ketones and does so efficiently without sugar.

With a liver that's firing on all four cylinders and a body that's burning ketones (optimally) you only need one more part to the puzzle. That final part is oxygen. With the liver working, starve the body of sugar, flood it with oxygen and good health can be yours for the taking! If you have the funds, flooding the body with oxygen is easy but I suspect not everyone who comes to this book has the means to pay for ozone therapy or a hyperbaric chamber (although I believe there are now companies online that rent chambers). Either way, in this internet savvy world, your options for increasing oxygen are plentiful.

While for legal reasons I cannot give you specific doses, I can at least suggest taking in an abundance of fresh air as a good starting point. Yup, there are a few other more controversial ways out there, but you should first consult with your doctor before attempting anything new.

A WHOLE NEW YOU

Give the body what it needs and it will find a way to renew itself. It's sometimes said that every seven years or so we grow ourselves a whole new body. While there is some truth to this concept, our cells are constantly replacing themselves at varying rates. The lining of the stomach, for example, is replaced about every three days, while it's estimated that bones turn over every seven to ten years. On average, the entire outer skin is replaced about every two weeks and the liver regrows itself every couple of years.

This cycle of events is not only remarkable it's a little freaky. Physically you are not the same person you were seven years ago. This presents a window of opportunity for anyone willing to make changes. How your body reacts tomorrow is closely tied to the raw materials being used today.

Even parts of your brain will regenerate, although not all. Some of us might warm to the idea of having a whole new brain; others will take comfort in knowing that essentially our memories remain the same.

As our time now draws closer to the end, I'm actually quite shocked at how much work goes into writing a book. Over the past year I've lost count of how many times I've had to dismantle this whole book and then rewrite it from scratch. When the madness of self-imposed standards met devotion, each and every paragraph became a bargaining chip for just a quiet moment alone with my own thoughts. To some degree, it's a relief to be almost at the finish line, but I'll also miss the process of writing for you as there was so much more I wanted to share.

So from here, I'm really not sure where I go next with my life. While construction work pays my rent, it really doesn't get any easier on the body. I guess a lot depends on whether this book strikes a chord with people. Unfortunately, the world has no shortage of struggling unknown authors. Perhaps I'll take out an ad in the local paper that reads, "Handyman – will write for food" lol.

What did we learn from this chapter?

Supermarket food is grown for profit. Those who eat it daily may at some point develop a mineral deficiency somewhere within the body.

Rapidly changing the gut biome can bring unwanted side effects. As always, go slow with a small test dose first rather than subjecting yourself to a mega dose. BEFORE moving into oral supplementation, try to gradually increase your probiotic intake through fermented foods.

Homework: check out a website by the name of earthclinic.com. It is full of helpful tips, all presented in an easy to understand format. It also covers supplements and a wide range of ailments. I use it often.

Link: https://www.earthclinic.com/

Could you please help me get to 100 reviews?

As we are now almost done with part 2 of this book, I'd be real interested to know how this information is being perceived. If you are enjoying it, please let me know. A one-line review on Amazon would be totally awesome. Doesn't have to be anything fancy, it could be just 5 words that say **"I enjoyed this book"** That's enough to let Amazon know this book has a value, which in turn helps to keep the book visible. Thank you in advance - *you know you rock right?*

Chapter 19

95% HOPE

As we now begin our final descent I'm reflecting on the time we have spent together. For a book written primarily about health it sure seems to have rendered its fair share of twists and digressions, and there are still a few more to come. At the beginning of this story you found me trapped inside a sickly body and unable to work. It's now been six years since I first became ill and seriously, as it happens and as I type this, it's actually six years to the day!

While I'm thankful for all the things I have learned, it might surprise you to know that I'd trade them all in a heartbeat not to have gone through what I did. Forgive me if I appear ungrateful, but clawing back 95% of my health isn't something I choose to celebrate. Nope, today's ironic anniversary is all about the 5% that's stubbornly remains, and how nobody has ever said "sorry."

Don't get me wrong, I'll take a partial recovery over no recovery any day of the week, but I'm also very aware that a problem left 5% unresolved is still a foot in the door to serious illness. I've worked hard to get to this point and yet there are days when trying to keep an annoying subset of rogue symptoms under my control feels as if I'm trying to hold a beach ball underwater. Here's one example.

Before I took my seat in that fateful doctor's office, running was something I took pleasure in. I could actually go quite a few miles without breaking a sweat. But once those unfortunate wheels were set in motion, things have never quite been the same and any attempt to run even a short distance still leaves my legs feeling heavy and tight. Rather than complain about it, I walk instead.

Given everything I was forced to learn and then apply, it's quite remarkable that this 5% still remains. I often wonder what would have become of me had I not been so persistent? What I do know for sure is this: whatever it was they introduced into my bloodstream in 2011, it still lurks inside me, albeit to a lesser degree.

Perhaps in this moment I'm seeing my glass as 5% empty, but so far I've narrowed it down to one of two things: either my own understanding of the problem has reached its limits, or the problem was intentionally made difficult to understand. If you choose to believe the latter, then it should also serve as a dark reminder that there are times when a routine doctor's visit can have destructive consequences.

Sometimes, the more you know, the more you wish you didn't know. As a direct result of that 2011 encounter, I've come to understand unless I find my silver bullet, my life may be shorter than even God intended. *I guess we will see.*

Those times when I've used the term "God" in this book it's been my feeble attempt to describe whatever entity governs this vast universe. I guess I find this concept more plausible that accepting we all somehow grew legs and walked ourselves out of the sea. History has a nasty habit of repeating itself and I suspect a day will come when science looks back on itself and asks, *what the hell were we thinking back in 2017?* The only thing we know for sure is that we are not the grand masters of the universe that we think we are.

That said, I'm really not a religious person either, but the day I felt the coldness of death moving through my bones I happened to come across a small piece of scripture that gave me a glimmer of hope. I'd like to share it with you because no matter *who* or *what* you believe in, when life gets too much to stand it sometimes helps to kneel.

"For I know the plans I have for you," declares the Lord,
"plans to prosper you and not to harm you,
plans to give you hope and a future."
– Jeremiah 29:11

When we are forced to accept our own mortality, what we choose to think has the power to enslave or liberate us on the turn of a single thought. Perhaps my eyes now see things differently. *How so?*

As someone who likes to be productive, the time I spent confined to a sick bed often left me feeling unproductive and isolated. In some ways, being trapped by illness gave me a rare insight as to how an inmate might cope when forced to endure a lifetime of incarceration. Sometimes the only places I got to visit were inside my head – barren destinations that frequently passed through my mind like tumbleweeds rolling across an open plain.

However, one place I visited was quite different, and to this day it's held a lasting impression. In the middle of enduring much suffering it was as if a gateway opened up deep in my subconscious. I can still recall in quite vivid detail standing barefoot inside a small stone cottage located somewhere on a grassy hill. The smooth stone floor warmed with the amber glow of sunshine which filtered through a stained glass window. I've never lived in such a place but it immediately felt like home and everything I touched had a distinct natural feel to it, almost as if plastic and paint had never been invented.

Within that fleeting moment of peace and simplicity it actually crossed my mind that perhaps my sickly body had given up and died. And to be honest, wherever it was that I'd found myself, I was in no rush to leave. Snapping back to reality left me reluctantly pondering the meaning of such a detailed image. Maybe I'd caught a glimpse of how we were supposed to live – in the moment, simply, and free of worry rather than chasing every dollar. I guess some parts of this book were inspired by that blissful feeling, others were written to address the inadequacies of a medical establishment that left me out to dry.

I know a solution is out there somewhere, but here I am still relying on persistence to find it. They say that persistence is believing that problems have solutions, just as doors have keys. It's the noble art of being knocked down ten times and getting up eleven. To be totally honest with you, my life is hard enough at the moment without getting knocked down. *I digress (often).*

So here we are at the end of the book, what say we drop it into four-wheel drive and go off road for a moment. Over the years I suspect you have had your fair share of troubles and I've had mine too. That ugly wheel of misfortune can be such an unpredictable part of life. We all have "character building" days – you know the ones I'm talking about, those days when you lose your job and your car keys in the same afternoon. Unfortunately, bad days aren't limited to losing replaceable things, although that sucks too.

Bad things happen to good people daily and none of us are immune. Maybe you already know what it's like to lose someone close to you, or perhaps you know what it's like to suffer from medical injury or be a victim of a crime. While our past certainly shapes us, it doesn't have to define who we are. For just a moment, I'd like to ask you to pause here, set down the book, and let your mind briefly drift back to one of those more challenging days.

I can only imagine where your mind went to and how that unfortunate day might have affected your life. I wonder, if you again had the opportunity to travel backward in time and were somehow able to stand next to yourself, what words of wisdom would you whisper in your ear?

For me, if I could go back in time, I'd tell myself, be still and know that in the end it's going to be okay. Just don't lose hope. In that hour of dark desperation, when a storm of shit seems to constantly rain down on us, we don't always need to know the reason; we just need to know it's going to be okay. It's as if our earthly soul needs something tangible to hold onto, perhaps just a small flicker of hope to reignite our human spirit. When we are deprived of such hope the world becomes a daunting place.

Understand that the vast majority of people on this planet all want the same things that you do, meaningful work, someone who believes in them, and *hope*. Nobody wakes up and asks, "How can I make my life more difficult today?" They really don't. No, that circumstance is usually imposed on us by the powers that be – but it doesn't have to be that way.

Look beyond those daily news headlines and you will notice that most of us are simply just trying to get by. Not everyone is an axe-wielding maniac, although there are some that are. Not everyone is out to deceive you, although there are some that will. It's my humble assumption that those who are exposed to a toxic environment are the ones mostly likely to make toxic choices.

Put your humanitarian goggles on for just a second and you will see that people are a product of their environment. You and I were not made to be dumb creatures. In case it escaped your attention, we are the *only* mammals on this planet driving around in cars, yet when the human brain is flooded with toxins we all have a tendency to make really dumb choices. Having seen a very different world, albeit briefly, I believe that simplicity is a greatly undervalued commodity and our world was never meant to be this toxic.

Alas, the darkness created in this life has always been rooted in greed and arrogance and yet it is this same darkness that helps us see the brightness of light.

You may have noticed how in recent times the word "hope" became part of a political slogan. The word was hyped up and bandied around with broad smiles and a promise that we all wanted to believe in. You may have also noticed political hope rarely reaches the bottomless pit of human despair. Stay with me here, because even though those damned spin doctors hijacked the word hope, it's vitally important they aren't allowed to keep it. *Come my friend, let us travel down one last road together.*

It's often said that gratitude can have a profound effect on the human soul. Gratitude has been shown to turn off stress, blast away critical thinking, wipe away selfishness, and even overturn that most destructive of all human conditions – victim mentality.

However, if you really want to take your health to a whole different level, learn to give and be grateful for the experience. I know what you are thinking because I thought it too – how much is this going to cost me, right? If counting your money with fingerless gloves on is your thang, then you can just go ahead and relax, this *final* health tip works with or without your money.

> To be truly radical is to make **hope** possible
> rather than despair convincing.
> – Raymond Williams

As rational thinkers, it can be difficult to understand how we can benefit ourselves by helping others. I wouldn't be wasting your time or mine if I hadn't experienced the value of this firsthand. Make no mistake, giving something back is a powerful tool to have under your belt. This can be as profound as saving a life or as simple as helping someone across the road. At this point, it's important not to let the simplicity of this concept undermine your perception.

Let's take a step back and look at this from a fresh angle. You can take it to the bank that right now there is someone out there who is experiencing a soul-crushing day, the depths of which you and I can only imagine. How would you like to become an intrinsic part of their story and in the process reap the reward? The trick to doing this is to expect nothing in return. Once you get to that level, something freaky happens. Giving freely opens the path to receiving. I know, right? But stay with me, I promise this final tip has a great deal of merit.

Back when I was too ill to work there were people in my local community who pitched in and left prepaid grocery and gas cards in my mailbox. Generosity came with no strings attached at a time when I felt had no value, although the money quickly came and went, those envelopes represented more than just food and gas, they also gave me **hope**. I later learned that some of those people who gave had never met me and yet they still chose to help. The fact that random people chose to step in without expecting anything in return kinda blew me away. Six years later those random acts of kindness remain firmly rooted inside me.

So where does all this fit in? Let's go back to that bad day you were having, maybe you did lose your car keys and your job in the same afternoon. On that lousy bus ride home how would you feel if suddenly you found an envelope on your seat. Inside that envelope there was no note, just a few dollars, perhaps only enough to buy yourself dinner at the end of a long miserable day. I know, right? WTF? (Who's-This-From?)

In the absence of any note you'd be forced to ponder the meaning of it all. Suddenly in the middle of a shit storm this becomes an almost surreal single ray of sunshine. But how the heck did that envelope find you on that bus, and why?

Here's how.

Whenever people stop what they are doing and take the trouble to look up from their phones, it becomes pretty easy to spot those around us who are having a really bad day – perhaps even struggling to keep their heads above water as I once was. To see someone who's genuinely in need and then, without drawing attention to yourself, be prepared to step in and help is a beautiful thing. But to anonymously put a few bucks in an envelope and find a way to discretely slip it to them becomes more than just a goodwill gesture, it's a symbol of hope.

Okay, where am I heading with all this?

There's a whole mountain of published scientific data that points to how we can lift ourselves by lifting others. No, seriously, this is sometimes referred to as **"Helper's-High."** One study showed that helping others led to a measureable increase in longevity (think of Edie Simms, that remarkable 102-year old lady who spends her days helping younger members of the nursing home!) Another study showed a measureable decrease in pain! With equal importance, it was also shown that people who observe feats of generosity are more likely to do the same, thus causing a ripple effect throughout an entire community. Wait a second, are you getting this? When one person performs a good deed, it literally causes a chain reaction of other altruistic acts!

The volume of data relating to this subject is incredibly vast, although it pains me to say I'm actually not a huge fan of citing scientific data. *Why?* Over the years I've lost count of how many times I've read something that was "cited" only to learn somewhere down the road that the data was skewed in favor of the person collecting it. But in this case there is no financial incentive behind the concept of giving freely, so the data is as pure as it can be! Don't take my word for it – if you like we can pause here while you go check it out even on sites such as PubMed.

Think about it, this world has become a breeding ground for habitual greed, egotism, and materialism and these are the very things that steal our inner peace. And most people don't even know it. The opposite end of that spectrum is to help someone and expect nothing in return.

To help you tap into the health benefits of this for yourself, it really doesn't matter what you do so long as you do it. Even if you don't have a spare dime, you can still get in the game by starting small, perhaps holding a door open for someone or simply making a conscious effort to let a few extra cars out in traffic. Over time you'll obviously want to step up your game, but for now it's all good. Notice that so far none of these ideas require large amounts of time or money.

If the secret to living is giving, then your mission from today on is a simple one: be a symbol of hope. Help someone, even in a small way, and in the process boost your own health!

So by making it this far you now have a comprehensive set of tools capable of bringing about a positive change. And (given the correct raw materials) you also have a body that knows how to heal itself.

As your new journey begins, treat these chapters as simple stepping stones and always be on the lookout for new and insightful information. These are exciting times we live in with fresh data constantly streaming in from every direction. Throughout this book I've always tried to keep things real. I've never pretended to have all the answers. I'm not sure anybody does. At best, discovery is a collective effort and a great starting point is to check out all those people mentioned by name in this book.

PERSISTENCE

With my story now drawing to a close, know that yours is just beginning. Over the course of this book we have crammed quite a few tools into our proverbial toolbox, and it seems that our old friend persistence remains a firm favorite, if for no other reason than it displays total disobedience in the face of adversity. Persistence lives deep inside each and every one of us, the trick is to bring it to the surface where it can be of most use to us.

Persistence requires no skill. It is nothing more than finding ways to move sideways when there appears to be no way forward. Persistence is simply about exhausting all options and then somehow finding a way to try just one more. It should come as no surprise that persistence is a close cousin of defiance. Once you have a handle on defiance you are rich for all that you need in this life.

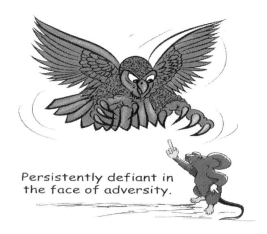

Persistently defiant in
the face of adversity.

Both persistence and defiance are such important qualities that I personally plan on taking them both with me to the afterlife. Prior to taking that great elevator to the sky, my last desperate breath on this earth will be spent trying to hold my middle finger in position. *Why?* "Victory belongs to the most persevering." - Napoleon Bonaparte. Besides, once rigor mortis sets in good luck to anyone attempting to straighten the finger out again! A little dark I know, but hey, given how ill I was back in 2011, I shouldn't even be here!

So until the day comes, I'll continue looking at my own health riddle objectively morning, noon, and night as I have done every day for the past six years.

As I write these final pages I'm also aware of how fickle the outside world can be, and perhaps I now set myself up for a few scathing reviews and even ridicule. I am at peace with this arrangement knowing that silence is a luxury best reserved for those unaffected by adversity. Fear of criticism is a poor excuse for not doing something. With that in mind, I find the words of Elbert Hubbard a comfort: **"To avoid criticism, do nothing, say nothing, and be nothing."**

Between books one and two, there are more than 142,000 words. I'm human, if any typos slipped through then I hope my passion for the subject will outshine my punctuation. Lord knows, trying to write out of a suitcase wasn't always easy, yet here we both are at the finish line.

I trust you have enjoyed reading this book as much as I have enjoyed writing it for you. Offering something safe and middle of the road was never my intention, and anything in between will surely have been a wasted effort. Maybe with more time, additional information could have been added but offering more would have also seen me teetering on the edge of procrastination and our paths might never have crossed. Creating something worthy of sharing was *always* my intended goal and it is my deepest hope that I have achieved that standard for you.

So before I crawl back under my rock, may I ask for a favor of you? With no slick, million-dollar marketing team behind me, good old fashioned word of mouth has always been my preferred way to advertise. If you enjoyed this book, would you please recommend it to a friend? As you probably guessed, marketing really isn't my thing, so I'll take all the help I can get. Your voice is my lifeline. A plug from you on any one the following platforms would be totally awesome.

☐ AMAZON
☐ GOODREADS
☐ FACEBOOK

For Amazon to sit up and take notice, this book needs at least a **100** reviews. As a struggling first time author, this presents a real challenge to me. *Your* review actually lets Amazon know that this book has a value. A simple one-line that says **"I enjoyed this book"** is perfect. I really appreciate your support, thank you.

As a passionate writer, it's still my dream to write full time. If given the opportunity, I'd like to share a lots of new topics that we simply didn't get time to cover in this book. I find depression and anxiety such fascinating topics and yet they are made so difficult for people to understand.

The challenge for me isn't finding things to write about, it trying to gauge when to stop, and tonight as I look up at the clock, here seems a good a place as any. So for now, I guess that's it, except to say thank you for your valued support and good luck on your own journey. Oh yeah, one last thing, **Dad, if you can somehow see me, I miss your face and I dedicate this book to you.**

Author gently sets down the pen and quietly leaves the room. I know, right? Dropping the mic would have been a tad pretentious.

Kindest Regards
James

A few photos follow, enjoy!

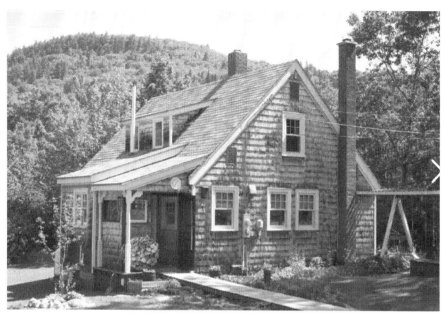

OUR OLD HOMESTEAD - NEW HAMPSHIRE

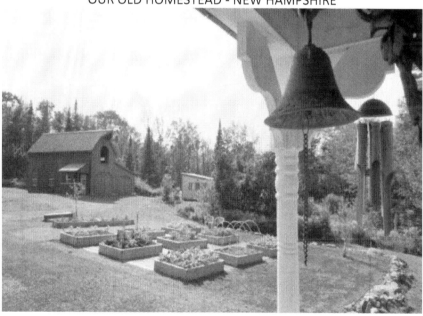

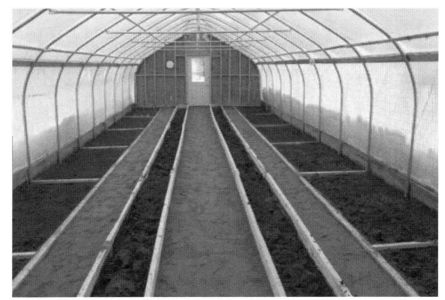

OUR OLD HOMESTEAD – NEW HAMPSHIRE

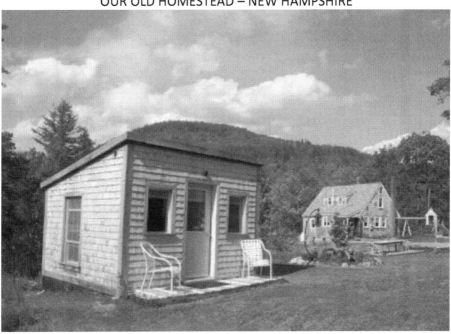

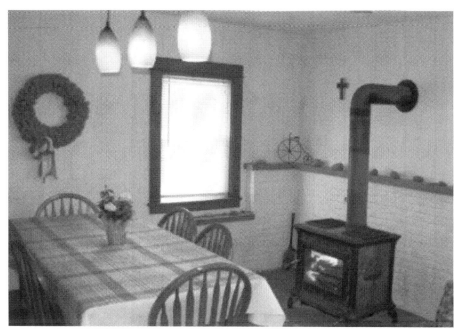

OUR SOLD HOMESTEAD - NEW HAMPSHIRE

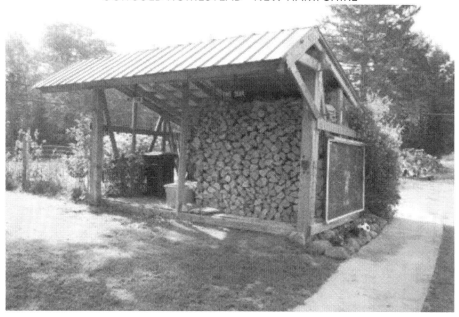

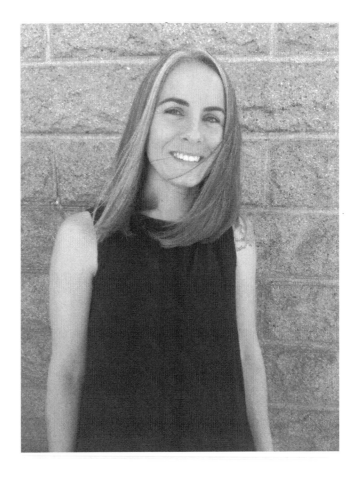

My wife Amanda, you can check out her
beautiful knitting patterns on Ravelry.com

Looking for a new place to call home.

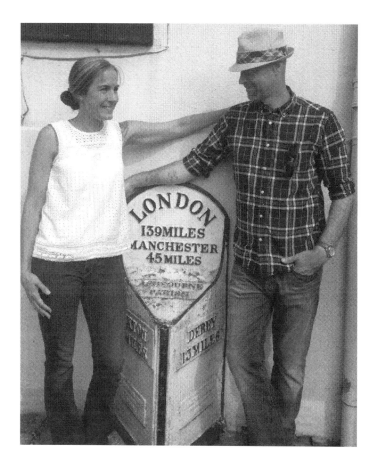

At the moment we haven't quite found a new place to call home, but you can tune in for updates by following us on Facebook

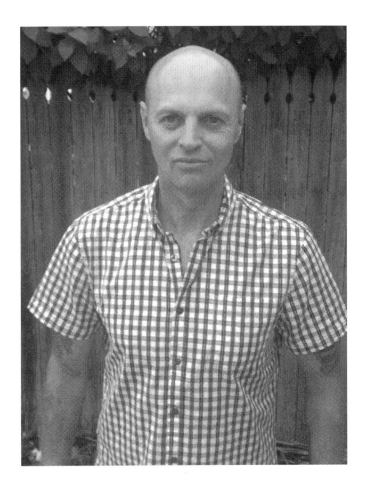

As someone who *dislikes* attention, I would rather not to have my photo taken. I'm here taking a hit for the team as a way of saying thank you to everyone, especially those people who took time out of their busy day to leave a review, **thank you.**

S.O.S
Would you please help me get to 100 reviews?

☆☆☆☆☆

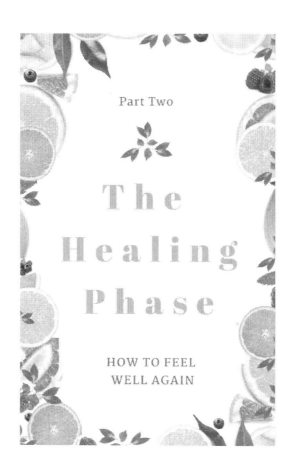

Part Two

The Healing Phase

HOW TO FEEL WELL AGAIN

A simple review that says
***"I enjoyed this book"* is perfect.**

Thanks for supporting an indie author,
I genuinely appreciate it.

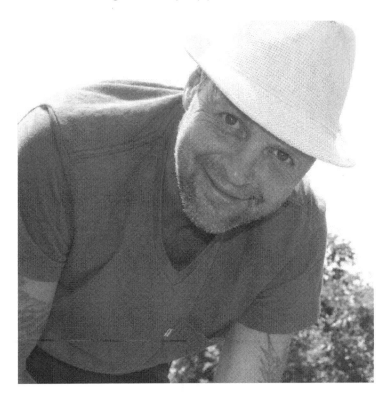

For fresh updates, come check out my Facebook page.

https://www.facebook.com/james.lilley.393950

SPECIAL THANKS TO

To my dear old mum, who I admire greatly. Standing at just 5ft 2, Jean is a woman of few words and not somebody you would want to mess with in a bar fight. I love her more than she will ever know, even though she watches violent cowboy movies while sucking loudly on extra strong mints.

My wife Amanda, I know this past year hasn't always been easy. Dealing with the madness of my new writing obsession while living on a shoestring budget was at times challenging. Perhaps now that the book is complete you can see why it was so important for me to finish. Thank you for always showing me what a PDF file is, I love you more than I love my new instant pot.

To my sisters, who over the years have always been so good to me, even though I happily drive them both bonkers. To Jade, you are stronger than you know and admire your spirit. To Cortney I genuinely apologize for messing things up. To the very unique Miss Emma, thank you for all your wonderful contributions to this book, your letter was quite moving. To the one and only Miss Abigail, thank you for always being you. For sure, Grandad would be so proud of you all.

To Derek Murphy, who very kindly gave up his valuable time to design this book cover without charge, (thank you so much). To Dalton Lawrence, thank you for your unwavering support, your true value in this life that has yet to be realized. To my old friend Steve Shaw, who is the 2nd best salesman I've ever met and whom I've always trusted to always tell me like it is. To my old army buddy Howie, stay safe and find peace. Thanks to to Kaylia Dunstan, thank you for helping to keep my thoughts on track.

For people who read from the back,
hello to you, *and here's what you missed.*

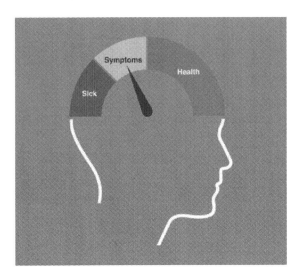

Based on six years of meticulous research, this remarkable 2-part story unfolds into a step-by-step, problem-solving tool. It's your shortcut to a less stressed, more energized, healthier version of you.

Here's what we know for sure.

In a perfect world a solution is found and once again life is good, but I'm guessing you already know the world we live in is far from perfect. What becomes of those who leave the doctor's office with a set of lingering symptoms, or a treatment plan that makes things worse? What's your next move if you are told your illness has no solution**? Do you have a plan?**

Come inside and discover the elusive answers you crave. Let the route to wellness take you down some beautiful winding roads. It's all in here waiting for you, peppered with a delicate hint of British humor.

Please share your story and become a part of it!

"I spent over an hour immersed in your book today, and am soooo grateful to you! Since beginning to implement things you've shared, I've cut my prescription down by 60%, and all of my levels have improved! I stopped using an acid reducing meds, my sugar consumption has drastically lessened, as has use of grains... it's a huge change, but it's getting easier as time goes on, and I'm starting to feel better... thank you, with all my heart!" - Teresa Blaisdell- NH

IF YOU LOVED IT,
THEN SET IT FREE!

And finally, I'd like to challenge you to set this book free. Leave a copy in the most random place you can think of perhaps with a five-dollar bill left inside as a bookmark. Let the finder experience a totally random act of kindness, and maybe in turn they will do the same.

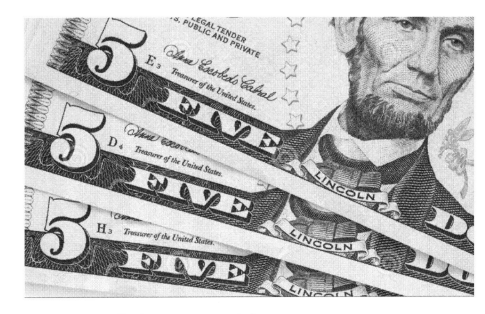

Feel free to send a photo of your liberated paperback to my FB page and I'll award a newly signed copy to the most interesting entry.
Be creative, be kind, be well.

Here's the link.
https://www.facebook.com/james.lilley.393950

Thank you
and Goodnight!

Printed in Great Britain
by Amazon